# Psychopathology and Religion

# Psychopathology and Religion

## Structural Convergences between Mental Disorders and Religion

Damian Janus
Translated by Barbara Gąstoł

LEXINGTON BOOKS
*Lanham • Boulder • New York • London*

Published by Lexington Books
An imprint of The Rowman & Littlefield Publishing Group, Inc.
4501 Forbes Boulevard, Suite 200, Lanham, Maryland 20706
www.rowman.com

6 Tinworth Street, London SE11 5AL, United Kingdom

British Library Cataloguing in Publication Information Available

**Library of Congress Cataloging-in-Publication Data**

Names: Janus, Damian, 1969- author.
Title: Psychopathology and religion : structural convergences between mental disorders and religion / Damian Janus ; translated by Barbara Gąstoł.
Other titles: Psychopatologia a religia. English
Description: Lanham : Lexington Books, [2019] | Includes bibliographical references and index.
Identifiers: LCCN 2018056261 (print) | LCCN 2018058691 (ebook) | ISBN 9781498578479 (Electronic) | ISBN 9781498578462 (cloth) Subjects: LCSH: Psychiatry and religion.
Classification: LCC RC455.4.R4 (ebook) | LCC RC455.4.R4 J3613 2019 (print) | DDC 616.89—dc23
LC record available at https://lccn.loc.gov/2018056261

# Contents

# Introduction

The book addresses the issue of relationships between psychopathological phenomena and religion. However, the work is more about psychopathology than about religion. A significant part of it is research, which can be described as phenomenology or hermeneutics of disorders. Therefore, it is not based on a simple scheme of juxtaposing knowledge in the field of religious studies with current psychiatric and psychoanalytic knowledge. Psychopathology is explicated here, in part, "in a new way," because certain disorders gain a new understanding, and commonly used psychiatric names are sometimes used only as waypoints or gateways to original reflections.

In the study, I search for the structures and mechanisms emerging in the course of mental disorders that have their counterparts in religiosity. I show that man is *homo religiosus* in a broad sense, because the processes of his mental life "give witness" to what religion emphasizes or tries to explain. Whereas the religious content can be regarded as a symbolic and synthetic depiction of the most important components of mental life. These identifiable factors, both within the framework of religion and mental disorders, seem to be relatively independent of social and historical conditions. As existential, they are constantly present in human life, playing a leading role in shaping the psychopathological image as well as in the genesis of religiosity (including fear of death, desire for power and lasting, need for predictability of life, need for care and other).

The book covers the topic of various mental disorders (neuroses, personality disorders, dissociative disorders, psychoses, eating disorders), symptoms (delusions, hallucinations, self-destructive behaviors), as well as the analysis of some more common psychological phenomena. It shows that mental mechanisms are often similar in cases of various disorders and syndromes, and even have their counterparts in the experiences we define as normal.

The book is based on my work as a clinical psychologist and psychotherapist in a psychiatric ward and private psychotherapeutic practice.

*Chapter One*

# Psychopathology and Religion: Towards the Non-Reductionist Approach

Motto:

*It is confessed that the utmost effort of human reason is to reduce the principles productive of natural phenomena to a greater simplicity and to resolve the many particular effects into a few general causes by means of reasonings from analogy, experience, and observation. But as to the causes of these general causes, we should in vain attempt their discovery, nor shall we ever be able to satisfy ourselves by any particular explication of them. These ultimate springs and principles are totally shut up from human curiosity and inquiry.* (Hume 2012, 844)

## WITELO—ONE OF THE PRECURSORS OF PSYCHOPATHOLOGY AND RESEARCH ON RELIGION

Witelo (ca. 1230–ca. 1314), the first significant Polish scientist, in the treatise *On the Nature of Demons*, wrote:

Some of them appear to those who suffer from dyscrasia and who are deranged by the pain born from an abscess of the meninges due to burning bile or the agitation of blood emitting hot fumes from the heart to the brain. Sometimes these phantoms are born from various sufferings, for example if the diaphragm, stomach, uterus, or any other part of the body rots, being at the same time connected to the brain through nerves. [. . .] then the sensory powers get into the brain, where the rational powers dominate and so the mental activities are stopped [. . .]. It is then that the power of the imagination is infected with sick (colored) images [. . .] which causes the imagination to forbid the higher, that is, mental, power to judge correctly [. . .] so that this higher mental power does not speak of real things, but considers images or ideas of things, and then, fantasizing itself, it judges fantasies. [. . .] And since every soul carries the reason for its fear with it, people are constantly in fear and say that they fear the demons, which they constantly see. (Witelo 2000, 33–34)[1]

Witelo, considered to be the pioneer of the scientific basis of optics—the author of *Perspectiva*, the work known in the Middle Ages (Trzynadlowski 1979; Dianni and Wachułka 1963, 23–28)—is also said to be the precursor of psychopathology (Burchardt 1979, 148–49). Interestingly, medical considerations in his treatise are closely connected to the demonological issues that were officially addressed by theology. Witelo admits, however, that he does not know theology and deals with the scientific side of the issue.

The author refers to two types of demons, the first of which is real beings, and the other—hallucinations. He argues that hallucinations result from—as we would now say—projections, i.e., from perceiving internal states as something external ("coloring the brain" with phlegm, bile, or blood). He points out that the cultural circle and the prevailing ideas have an influence on the interpretation of hallucinations—where someone from one culture recognizes a demon, a member of another culture may see an angel. Delusions—as we refer to these products now—are formed because the mind draws conclusions not on the basis of observations but imaginations (hallucinations). Witelo claims that hallucinated demons do not affect the external world in any way, but he admits that these hallucinations can affect the human organism. This influence occurs because the soul, changing itself, also changes the body. Witelo—to use contemporary language—describes psychosomatic reactions. He also says that "every soul carries the reason for its fear with it" (Witelo 2000, 34), so he recognizes psychological sources of anxieties.

Speaking of the basis of hallucinations in terms of brain pathology, organ diseases, and imbalance of humors, Witelo takes a stance close to the biomedical approach, according to which mental disorders result from somatic pathology. However, when he additionally states that the "rational soul" in epileptics and apoplectics—physically ill, by the way—may separate from the senses and return to the eternal, "omniscient substance," which makes them able to foretell the future, he admits that people suffering from mental disorders may open to something that they would not be aware of in a normal state. Thereby, he is close to the view of contemporary transpersonal psychology.[2]

## PSYCHOPATHOLOGY AND
## RELIGION—TYPES OF RELATIONS

There are three major approaches to the issue of relations between religion and mental disorders. The first one sees religious phenomena as forms of mental disorders. Religious phenomena are analyzed in the framework of psychiatric or neurophysiological conceptualization and are reduced to psychopathological phenomena. So it is a reductionist approach. It is within this approach that claims are made that possession is nothing but hysteria and that mystical states result from psychasthenia (Wulff 1999, 50–54). The reductionistic approach is often equated with the scientific approach, as reductionism is an important methodological element of science. However, although it triumphed in the natural sciences, the human sciences obviously point to its limitations. It entails the tendency to simplify—to make a religious phenomenon fit the psychopathological pattern, one often fails to notice those aspects of it that do not match the pattern. Of course, this attitude, apart from drawbacks, has also merits. During the development of witchcraft trials (sixteenth–seventeenth centuries), a scientific discussion was started on how mental illnesses could affect alleged witchcraft activities, irrespective of the devil's possible influence, or lack thereof (Levack 1991, 69–72; Trillat 1993, 30–42). This type of reduction of "supernatural" states to mere madness was certainly not a negative process. Especially for the accused.

The second standpoint is the opposite; it analyzes psychopathology with the help of religious ideas, for example, it explains psychological disorders in the light of Christian theology. Those who adopt this approach do not try to explain religion, but rather psychological disorders. Things like the existence of God, spirits, and angels are quite obvious to its representatives. For them, only the causes and functions of mental disorders need to be explained. In the simplest, even primitive view, the disorders can be perceived as punishment for sins sent by God. They can also result from an impersonal mechanism, which causes that certain acts or transgressions of principles lead to psychological problems. This understanding is specific to the concept of Hindu karma. A disease can also be related to the interactions of the human soul with the souls of other people, ghosts, and demons. Some contemporary exorcists claim that even behaviors and symptoms like compulsive onanism or promiscuity arise from the influence of the "demon of impurity." There are also psychotherapists who argue that various disorders of their patients result from the influence of "lost souls" of the deceased that "attach" to the psyche of the living (Fiore 1995).

Madness itself, since it was considered to be connected with the sacred, was valued not only negatively. In antiquity, attempts were made to identify diseases with both natural and god-derived processes, including, for example, epilepsy called the divine disease (Bednarczyk 1999, 168 et seq.). Plato, through the mouth of Socrates, says:

> For if it were simply the case that madness is something bad, it would be beautifully said; but as things are, the greatest of good things come into being for us

through madness, when, that is, it is given with a divine being. For the prophet-
ess in Delphi and the priestesses in Dodona when mad have accomplished many
beautiful things for Greece both in private and in public, but little, or rather
nothing, when of sound mind. (Plato 1998, 47)

Does the discussed approach to the relationship between religion and psychopathology—as it seems completely outdated—have any value? Yes, because it suggests that mental disorders may be associated with a wider background than the one modern psychiatry suggests, reducing them to purely
physical brain disorders. After all, pointing to such "pathogenic" factors as
guilt, sin, transgression against natural or divine law broadens the perspective
on mental disorders, connecting them with the manifestations of our spiritual
life, and not only with the physiology of the brain.

The third possible stance would consist in disconnecting the issues of psychopathology from religious life and analyzing them separately. According to
this approach we would need to assume that mental illnesses have nothing to
do with the spiritual world, and "genuine" religious phenomena are certainly
not products of a disturbed psyche. This approach would obviously not contribute to the development of the understanding of the relationship between
the psyche and religion. Adopting this position, we would have neither the
motivation nor the possibility of building new knowledge in the field. The
psychological functioning of man would not teach us anything about religiosity, and religions would not tell us much or anything about the psyche.
This stance is represented by many contemporary Christians, who want to be
considered rational, as well as by Christian psychiatrists, who think that mental disorders are common diseases, from which they exclude possession as a
purely religious phenomenon that has nothing to do with psychopathology.

## Reductionism and Biomedical Understanding of Mental Disorders

In science, the most common way to connect religion and psychopathology
is to adopt the reductionist position. One tries to explain religions, which are
mysterious and heterogenic phenomena, by reducing them to psychopathological phenomena that are considered to be simpler and more understandable. Why? It seems that it is easier to regard religion—its genesis, essence,
and meaning—as a matter that is mysterious and difficult to understand than
to admit that mental disorders are equally mysterious and not fully examined.
After all, the psychiatrist *knows* the latter, he constantly deals with them,
cures them. They are only a group of more or less chaotic malfunctions of
people's thinking, behavior, and emotional life. So if a disorder is something understandable for a biologist, physiologist, or physician, it can be
used to explain other phenomena, which are found less obvious. When we

regard a given religious phenomenon as a result of—approached this way—pathology, it also becomes ordinary and scientifically controlled.

However, mental disorders do not have to be so simple. They seem to be like this only when we adopt the biomedical disease model. According to this model, mental illnesses (mental disorders) have the same status as somatic diseases—they amount to a certain disturbance in normal functioning. This model assumes that the basis of mental disorders is the body (brain, neurotransmitters, neurophysiology, genes). The biomedical model of mental disorders developed as part of treatment of somatic diseases associated with physiological research, pharmacotherapy, hospitalizations, and the authoritarian approach to patients. It has very serious consequences in the form of preferred treatment methods, ways of informing and cooperating with patients' families, adopting certain legal solutions, and—perhaps most importantly—dealing with patients.[3] Even referring to mental problems as "disorders" or "diseases" reveals the impact of this model. It simply seems that—as in this work—we cannot avoid its influence speaking of "psychopathology." It is one thing to use medical tradition, it is quite another to blindly believe in the complete correctness of this model.

If we allow ourselves to be unbiased and open, we can easily see that mental disorders are very different from somatic diseases, and that the biomedical model is not adequate here. The main difference is that mental disorders relate to the sphere that cannot be objectified. These disorders are "mental," which means that they occur in the area called "subjective" or "internal," as opposed to the objective external world. We never have full access to mental disorders from the outside, and to study them, we must not disregard the patient as a subject. In other words, there is no objective psychiatric examination. We often hear that someone is "admitted to observation," "subjected to psychiatric examination," etc. These wordings suggest that "mental health" can be examined objectively. This is a falsification of the actual state. Of course, the psychiatrist performs an examination—usually based on a conversation consisting of a template set of questions—but the conclusions he may reach are very general and influenced by his own ideas. The status of such an examination is completely different from the status of the tests conducted in the case of somatic medicine, such as an ECG.

Yes, there are also some instrumental ways to approach the individual's internality. These can be psychometric tests, neurological reflex tests, electroencephalography, computer brain imaging, hormone and neurotransmitter tests, or eye movement analysis. These methods can give us a picture of "character traits," "symptoms," "mechanisms," can suggest a likely course of the "disease" and possible types of help. However, they never really reach the subjective area, the area of the subject. In order to get closer to it, we must treat the patient in the same way as we treat our friends when we want to get to know them better. We do not force our friends to answer, nor do we try to look into their windows to find out how they are. We rather gain their trust and talk to them. This means treating the patient as a subject. The biomedical approach tries to avoid it, and that is why it cannot get to know the functioning of the psyche more deeply.

A disease brings suffering, which is why it may seem to us that the prevailing model of disease, as something exclusively evil and unnecessary, is obvious. When we suffer from a somatic disease, we want the condition from before the disease back, as we remember it as a state of harmony and peace. The disease is perceived as a kind of ulcer that needs to be removed to make the tissue healthy again. This pattern is quite adequate in relation to many somatic disorders; however, transferred to the ground of mental problems, it fails almost completely. One can easily see that the understanding of the disease must be different in these two cases. A person who is infected or affected by genetic defects may be perceived as suffering from something that is completely independent of him. Is it the same with neurosis? It seems otherwise. After all, it occurs in the same "place" where our identity "resides," in the psyche. Thus, a mental disorder is always "more me," "more under my influence," "closer to my personality" than a somatic disease.

In the case of more serious dysfunctions, such as psychoses, the objectifying biomedical model may seem more adequate (and sometimes it is, for example in cases of brain inflammation, its injury, intoxication, etc.). In contact with a psychotic person, we may have the impression that he is completely "overwhelmed by the sickness," that basically there is no subject any longer. That there is nobody to talk to. That there is only the disease. However, if we see the patient this way, we can use the procedures that we consider to be objectively healing without considering the world of the sufferer's experiences. In this way, four paramedics can, without trying to calm the frightened patient through talking to him, immobilize him and strap him to the bed in order to pharmacologically heal his anxiety, ignoring the fact that through this action, the anxiety will intensity. In reality, however, when we approach the patient with sufficient patience, it turns out that even in severe psychoses there is a subject. His world has become completely alien to the social world. However, it is a certain world and a certain way of being, not just a tangle of irrelevant things. Only an external, impatient observer believes it to be so.

However, in the biomedical model, there is no room for the hypothesis that psychotic thinking may be sensible or that psychosis may have some developmental aspects. Similarly, there is no room in it for any extraordinary experiences of healthy people. This model separates the sick from the healthy, and if the latter display something unusual, for example, claim that they are clairvoyant, they are suspected of being mentally ill. The model introduces a vision of "mentally healthy" people and "diseases" that lie in wait for them. It also implicitly suggests that both of these elements are basically known—both "people" and their "illnesses." In fact, it is not at all clear what the healthy psyche is or what mental disorders mean in our lives. We only have a very imperfect model that turns out to be deficient in far too many cases.[4]

The concept of illness derived from somatic medicine seemed to be able to reduce various mental phenomena to "nothing more than diseases." However, what we call a disease seems so simple just because we have created a simple model. The true attitude of the subject to the disease, the relationship of man and his problem, is not at all simple and has not been explained. Pathology of the psyche is no less incomprehensible than the psyche in general. So if we continue to try to reduce religious phenomena to psychiatric problems (for example, claim that experiencing presence of the deceased must be psychosis), we are at risk of making the *ignotum per æque ignotum* error, explaining the unknown by the equally unknown.

## OBJECTIVISM AND CONSTRUCTIVISM

There are—in my opinion—two basic approaches to knowledge, two kinds of status we attribute to it. Adopting one or another of them has far-reaching consequences. Our approach to knowledge results in the way we use it and, as a consequence, do our work (for example as a physician or psychotherapist), it also translates to our worldview, and the way we live. I define these two different attitudes as objectivism and constructivism. I do not think that choosing one of them is generally fully deliberate. On the contrary, I think that it is usually unreflective, especially when it comes to following the objectivist stance that seems to be more commonsensical. I will now discuss both of these perspectives.

Objectivism exalts the status of our knowledge. Knowledge, a statement about reality, becomes absolutized, considered to be, in a way, reality itself. I believe this approach dominates in science. It regards knowledge of reality as a collection of some kind of "objects." In this approach, words (signs, codes) seem to directly correspond with things, somehow contain them. They become not only a sign of things, but even a copy of them. Let us think about physics. Mathematical constructs replace reality in it. This is, of course, fully justified, because only a mathematical apparatus allows to carry out new, and consistent with the previous, reasoning, so that it is possible to predict the results of future experiments. However, the "change" of reality for mathematics is not fully legitimate from the ontological point of view. Recently, for example, string theory develops, in which "strings" are the smallest "building blocks" of reality. Physicists imagine that at a fundamental level the world is built of "vibrating strings." However, ontologically, one can be sure that the world *is not* made of strings. Strings are only mathematical idealizations and, in part, products of our imagination. We cannot see anything else, but it does not mean that there is nothing else. The proof that there is always *something more* is on the one hand the series of idealizations and abstractions to be carried out in order to achieve a coherent vision, such as string theory, and, on the other, constant variability of our knowledge and theories.

In biology textbooks we can find simple principles of inheritance according to the laws formulated by Gregor Mendel. Everything is transparent and presented as numerical relationships. It seems that the Augustinian showed us the almost mathematical foundation of the reproduction of organisms. As if there were a few core rules behind all the variability and exuberance of life. And it is so. However, only through idealization. It has been known for some time now that Mendelian rules do not always apply (Spork 2011, 274). It is similar in every science and in every theory—sooner or later it turns out to be an approximation of reality, not its essence. This happened, for example, with Newton's mechanics, which was supposed to represent the iron laws of the universe, and turned out to be only their imperfect approximation, in the face of the fuller view of gravity presented by Albert Einstein. This is also clearly visible in medicine. Free radicals damaged cells, so they had to be neutralized with antioxidants. The dependency relationship seemed simple. Later, however, the picture became more complex and free radicals turned out to be important signaling factors, involved, for example, in the work of the heart. Similarly, in many cases, when we examine matters closer, the picture becomes more complicated, revealing a whole bunch of previously unnoticed dependencies. Is the new image final? Of course not, because science is constantly evolving. Is the new image sometimes less complicated than the old one? No, everything tends to be more complex. What is the conclusion? That the universe has always something to hide, that processes we do not see yet constantly occur.

Take the following example to illustrate simplifying tendencies in our thinking. Imagine a device such as a television set. It is an object made of electronic components connected according to a certain diagram. If we familiarize ourselves with the elements and the diagram, we can say that we *have known* it. The entire television set is defined by the type of *elements* and the *diagram* used. Can we think about man in a similar way? Yes, we can say that the human body *consists of* the nervous, circulatory, skeletal, respiratory, and other systems. The nervous system is *built from* neurons and other tissues from different cells. It seems, then, that one can speak of the elements and the scheme of their order also in relation to man. There is a subtle distinction: the nervous, blood and any other systems do not build a person as such but the "man-we-know." This "man" is never a "real" man but a theoretical reconstruction, created within a given state of culture and science. How can we tell that man as such and the man known to science differ? For example, by the fact that the course of physiological processes, diseases, or reactions to negative factors is different in different people and often significantly deviates from the standards described in medical textbooks. We know well how often physicians are wrong in their prognoses and opinions. This is because there are processes and structures unknown to current medicine.

Knowing how a television set is *built* seems to be more complete than knowing the structure of man: knowing the structure of a television set, we can construct it; knowing the structure of a living organism, we are not able to do it. However, in both cases the limitations of our knowledge are in fact similar. Even a thing like a television set, although created by us, is unknown to us at the same time. It may seem simple if we are satisfied with just the model that only describes electronic components and their arrangement. However, transistors are made of some kind of material, which consists of different substances, these in turn consist of molecules that are built from particles of matter. And what is matter? Has it revealed all its secrets to us? From this perspective, we do not know everything about our television set. The electronics engineer assembling the device does not analyze this, letting thousands of phenomena take place without his knowledge. And yet he claims that he *knows* the structure of the device. His cognitive attitude that the transistor is "just a transistor" protects him from an outburst of questions and uncertainties. Are scientists, even physicists studying matter alone, not like electronics engineers? They also have to assume "obviousness." For each science creates compact "blocks," schemes it does not further analyze. But apart from diagrams, formalisms, models, and theories, something still remains—active reality, permanently intangible in its entirety.

Most scholars seem to be immersed in objectivism. Although they accept the obvious fact that science develops and that we have not learned everything yet, they tacitly assume that many aspects of the world have been thoroughly examined. One cannot agree with that. Looking at our knowledge with greater deliberation, considering the change in scientific theories, the area of the unknown, as well as any anomalies (medical, psychological, cosmological), we must come to the conclusion that only our models can be simple and obvious, while phenomena always show a specific depth. And here the constructivist stance,[5] as I understand it, emerges. This attitude consists in being aware of the difference between reality and the concepts and theories on it. In short, we recognize the existence of the mystery and the unknown in the world. The point is to realize that we do not even know what we have already known and that the world is more complicated than our understanding of it.

The constructivist stance has its precursors in Greek atomism, represented by Democritus, who said, "By this principle [atomism] man must know that he is removed from reality" (quoted in Taylor 2003, 229), and in the attitude of the skeptics, who ordered to refrain from unambiguous judgments about things. Later, particularly David Hume pointed to our tendency to overestimate our own knowledge. This is well illustrated by his analysis of the causal relationship (see Hume 2012, 851 et seq.). Hume shows that having access only to the correlations between phenomena, we have an irresistible impression of the existence of fundamental relations, such as the cause-and-effect relationship. It seems to us that causality objectively exists, but in reality we are influenced by the mental process. In a sense, we see a "tappet" that goes from the cause and meets the effect. Thus, we simplify nature, guided by a subjective sense of simplicity and obviousness. Again, in place of reality, we insert a diagram.

Immanuel Kant also tried to separate what exists from what we know (Höffe 1995, 132–34). Kant's reasoning is elaborate and cannot be fully reconstructed here. According to the philosopher, all knowledge emerges in the process of a kind of projection of our mental categories onto the outside world. However, this world exists also regardless of the cognitive activities of man. Kant referred to this foundation of knowledge, which, however, we cannot directly access, as the "thing-in-itself." Everything we have learned is the result of its impact on our senses and mind, thus reality does not seem to be limited only to these mental representations.

A critical view of human cognition as unable to capture "reality," but conditioned by the social, historical, psychological, or biological context is advocated by Thomas Kuhn (Kuhn 2012), Humberto Maturana (Maturana 1998), or the so-called Edinburgh School, whose exponent, David Bloor claims that "Knowledge [. . .] is better equated with Culture than Experience" (Bloor 1991, 16). The fact that individuals nurse such and no other beliefs stems from the necessity to participate in social communication, the social context affects what we perceive in the world and what we consider to be knowledge. The above concepts, although very different, indicate that reality, whatever it is, does not impose unambiguous representations in the mind that is an active and creative factor.

There is no one constructivism, and the concept can be understood in many ways. The constructivism I propose emphasizes not knowledge, but ignorance. At the same time what we do not know is not nothingness. The processes unknown to us are active in the world. However, we always have only our concepts, diagrams, and theories concerning reality. Of course, in a sense, they give us access to it, but they never allow us to fully understand and master it. They are like reins that usually allow one to control the horse, but whose movements and stresses do not give a full picture of what a horse is.

Constructivism will then mean feeling the distance between our simplifying concepts and the complex reality. Our awareness of the split, or gap, changes our attitude towards knowledge of the psyche, psychology, psychoanalysis, psychiatry. It changes the understanding of mental illnesses, and consequently affects the style of the physician's or therapist's contact with patients. It allows a more open attitude towards everything that we encounter in the world of human experiences and problems. We do not have to immediately classify or "understand" these things, knowing that they certainly have their own depth. If psychology does not know and even cannot know who man is, then each of our encounters with a patient potentially puts us in a situation of discovering unknown aspects of the psyche.

The researcher whose reasoning is closest to mine is Ludwik Fleck (Fleck 1979).[6] Fleck was a microbiologist who also studied the history and philosophy of science. He showed how much a scientific fact, which seemingly is determined only by objective reality, depends on the cultural context, which Fleck referred to as a thought style. Fleck presented the sociological and cultural determinants of the concept of syphilis and Wassermann reaction, as it would seem, unambiguous scientific facts. Thus, he revealed the imperfection of the concepts of "objective reality" and an "objective fact." According to the title of his book, a scientific fact arises and develops and is not simply a reflection of the present "reality" (Fleck 1979). Another thing is also important in Fleck's reasoning. Above, I wrote that it is obvious that there are processes in the world that we do not know *yet*. But constructivism, as I understand it, also allows the possibility—and we have the premises, studying, for instance, ancient methods of treatment, such as acupuncture—that there are phenomena we *no longer* understand. Due to a certain development of culture and science, the concept of the four elements does not make sense to us any longer, and our Western medicine cannot find links between meridians and what it believes is important here; that is, the nervous system.

## PSYCHOTHERAPY, PHENOMENOLOGY, HERMENEUTICS

Examining mental life and its pathology, I adopted the hermeneutic attitude that is also close to phenomenology. I tried to apprehend the phenomena without excessively employing the psychiatric or psychoanalytic theories. At the same time, I investigated them in a wider context, and tried to present one narrative for psychological and psychopathological processes as well as certain phenomena and ideas in the field of religion or philosophy. The hermeneutic approach adopted here consists in finding connections of the studied area with the widest available background. My point was to consider pathological phenomena and "normal" human experiencing on a common plane (Laing 1999, 39 et seq.), to search for meaning in the disease, as well as "abnormality" in everyday life.

The data presented in this work is based on the observation of patients, or, more precisely—conversations being part of their psychotherapeutic processes. It is not just the observation "from the outside," but also empathizing with the patient. This or other "empathizing" or being induced in a therapeutic situation has a long tradition in psychoanalysis. Starting from Sigmund Freud's notion of "evenly-suspended attention" ("free-floating attention"), through his statements on the need to open the therapist's unconscious to the patient's unconscious and terms such as countertransference or projective identification, psychoanalysis in various ways has acknowledged the fact that in a therapeutic situation the therapist's mind functions in a specific way, being in an unusual connection with another person, which is unobservable in everyday life. This also involves intuition that allows one not to get lost among the multitude of material that patients bring and to extract the most important things. Intuition makes it possible to synthesize the information and reach a conclusion that would not be available in a purely rational way of thinking (Horney 2000, 72–75).[7]

Psychotherapy does not need to be only a treatment method, but is also a specific research methodology.[8] Cognition obtained on this path is impossible to achieve through another research procedure (e.g., psychological experiment, questionnaire and statistical analysis, interviews, psychophysiological and other tests). The information that opens up before the psychotherapist, focused on his patient's words and experiencing for months or years, is inaccessible to another researcher. A long time spent in psychotherapeutic sessions cannot be bypassed by any technical procedure, from psychological tests to hypnosis.

Relevant information about the patient is not available in his memory, like in a computer database. At the beginning of therapy, much of this information simply does not exist. It does not exist in verbal form. Man does not carry all of his history in the form of sentences. The most important mental processes are not available to the consciousness. They often reveal themselves only in an interpersonal relationship. In a therapeutic relationship, the patient not only *talks about* himself, but also *shows* himself. The literal content of the patient's communication is only a small part of what is important. Therapeutic work is mostly reading between the lines.[9]

## RELIGIOUS ELEMENTS IN PSYCHOPATHOLOGY

Religious elements in mental disorders can be identified in three forms, namely as: (a) belonging to the picture of the disease, explicitly expressed sentences of religious nature or such behaviors; (b) statements and pathological behaviors that, even if they do not directly address religious content and do not concern the sphere of religion, seem to be conditioned by religious culture; (c) systems of behavior, thoughts, and ideas presented in the context of mental disorders that do not have their direct and primary source in the impact of religious culture, but their form resembles some religious phenomena.

Point (a) relates to the phenomena in which the pathoplastic influence of religious content co-creates the picture of mental disorder. This is particularly vivid in the course of disorders called by psychiatry with a general name of schizophrenia. I mean different kinds of delusions or hallucinations of the religious nature. The elements distinguished in point (b) are particularly evident in neuroses. The form and intensity of the pathological sense of guilt, sexual fears, immature morality based on the message from external authority figures, and other aspects of psychopathology of neuroses of this type may be associated in many ways with the influence of religious culture. Point (c) identifies disorders whose course—understood as a complex of behaviors and thoughts, ideas, and tendencies—seems to be somewhat parallel to certain ways of functioning and experiencing of a religious man. Examples are rituals of obsessive-compulsive disorder and anorexia nervosa, in the course of which a characteristic pattern of functioning arises—a sick girl in a more or less conscious way "rejects" her body, associating it with danger and evil. Thus, she has an attitude similar to that of religious ascetics.

It should be noted that these three planes are not separable, and ascribing them to respective disorders is only relative. For example, obsessive-compulsive disorder, as structurally convergent with religious rituals, falls under point (c), although it may display the elements described by point (a), occurring in the form of religious behaviors (e.g., obsessive blasphemous thoughts or compulsive "crossing oneself"); its development can also result from strict religious education, which would mean that point (b) also plays a part here.

Religion and pathology are regular elements of life in all civilizations and cultures, and the capability of religious experiencing and susceptibility to pathological reactions are specific to man. Psychopathology, revealing the mechanisms of the psyche, also shows its "pro-religious" dimensions, man's natural readiness for religiosity. Looking from this perspective, I try to describe the phenomena similar to those that Bronisław Malinowski called "elementary acts of faith" (Malinowski 1984, 120). Malinowski denied that religious beliefs result from the work of the intellect, claiming that in man there is yet another plane which, irrespective of reason, shows us the existence of things. This emotional level constantly implies that there is something to believe in that the intellect "does not believe in." Kicking the stone one has nearly tripped over can be an example. Malinowski does not belittle the process that occurs in such a case, he does not say, for instance, that it is "only temporary emotions." Instead, he states that in such moments we produce a kind of faith. In this case, we personify the stone, "we believe" that it can spite us.[10] Similarly, when in the dark, we turn with horror towards the direction of the rustle we have just heard. When frightened, we believe in ghosts for a split second. Thus, the content of beliefs can—as Malinowski says—be created from nothing, or, more precisely, from the nature of our emotions. The researcher wrote:

> To argue the scientific stance adopted here, one should consider, from our point of view, the whole range of emotional life on the one hand—and the whole range of religious beliefs and practices on the other, and show how far the relationship between these two factors reaches and where it manifests. (Malinowski 1984, 133)[11]

In this book, I follow this idea and based on observations in the field of psychopathology, I show the variety of mental life and its connections with religion. What I present, corresponds with Mircea Eliade's statement that man is *homo religiosus*, as well as with Carl Gustav Jung's thesis that the soul is religious by nature (Jung 1999, 24–25). Jung wrote about the "religious function" of the soul ("soul"—the whole of the conscious and unconscious psyche), which means that its structure—manifested in dreams, visions, and other elements of mental functioning—corresponds with the universal religious images. Jung's work shows that the better we know the psyche, the more themes, images, and religious content we encounter; and the more we get to know religions, the more chance we have to understand the functioning of the psyche.

Perhaps the course of schizophrenic psychosis in a specific way indicates the fundamentality of the religious aspect in our lives. The expressions of many schizophrenics concentrate on religious, eschatological, and metaphysical issues (Kępiński 1992, 132–37). It is as if the disorder revealed inherent metaphysical and religious questions of every human being.

Having the influence of culture and social context in mind, we must not, of course, see what occurs in psychosis as a kind of *lingua naturalis*, a clear manifestation of the religion-forming forces in man. It seems, however, that since the issue of religion occurs so regularly in psychosis, it must emerge from the very foundation of mental life. Specific religious contents that schizophrenic patients manifest must result from cultural transmission, but the strength of the patients' religious commitment and their ability to create their own religious contents indicate that the predisposition to religiosity is an important element of the mental equipment of man. This is true despite the fact that religious themes may have a defensive function against the basic drive conflict, that is, serve as masking or mediation elements, or as means of expression. Religion is not just an external product to the soul, reaching it only through social interactions, but somehow corresponds, in its content and structure, to the depths of the psyche.

## NOTES

1. Quotation translated from Polish by Barbara Gąstoł.

2. Transpersonal psychology points to the factors of psychological life that go beyond the individual biography and perception (Drury 1995). In this approach mental problems may disrupt social adaptation, but they can support one's development in terms of his broader, "cosmic" personality. In Poland, Kazimierz Dąbrowski, using the concept of "positive disintegration," made an effort to show the positive aspects of mental disorders (Dąbrowski 1979).

3. An ex-patient, Dorothea Sophie Buck-Zerchin, writes about the negative consequences of the biomedical disease model: "Throughout medicine, there is no theory that has had such a disastrous effect on us, the persons affected by psychiatry, as the 'medical disease model' of [. . .] genetic and physical, [. . .] endogenous psychoses, especially schizophrenia. Because it prevents any dialogue about the contents of psychoses and their correlations with the previous life crises of those affected; because it attributes the highest therapeutic value to psychotropic drugs, although they can only suppress symptoms, but cannot heal; because it deprives those affected of the meaning of their particular emotional experiences and thus their development potential; because it blocks the self-help forces and discourages those affected instead of encouraging them. The 'medical disease model' tempts biologically oriented psychiatrists to explain to their patients that they suffer from 'incurable schizophrenia' and therefore need to take medication all their lives. This daunting prospect that one will be stigmatized for life as an 'incurable schizophrenic' and have to take medications that negatively influence feelings and initiative has already led far too many to suicide" (Buck-Zerchin 2000, 186; quotation translated from Polish by Barbara Gąstoł).

4. The theory of salutogenesis presented by Aaron Antonovsky does not recognize the dichotomy of "health/disease," but suggests a continuum whose extremes are purely theoretical (Antonovsky 1995, 19 et seq.). According to this author, a disease is no exception but a norm of the life process. Everyone is in part "sick" and although he may move towards the pole of "health," he will never reach it. This stance is opposite to the pathogenetic approach that prevails in medicine, which seeks "pathogenic factors" disrupting the state of homeostasis, harmony, and health considered to be the basic human condition.

5. Capturing the meaning of the discourse presented here is of fundamental importance for the understanding of the nature of delusions I address in the chapter on schizophrenia. It is also important for understanding of obsessive-compulsive disorder, and for analyzing the relationship between theological visions and psychopathological theories in the context of research into possession.

6. Ludwik Fleck (1896–1961), Polish microbiologist and philosopher of Jewish origin. He initiated the constructivist sociology of knowledge, and his concepts anticipated Kuhn's commonly known notions.

7. Einstein claimed that the basis of his creative thinking was not a language understood in a common way, not even a mathematical apparatus, but rather a kind of kinesthetic, bodily thinking (Sacks 1998, 66–67). I would define the intuition that I know from my own experience just as kinesthetic.

8. Freud writes: "In psychoanalysis there has existed from the very first an inseparable bond between cure and research. Knowledge brought therapeutic success. It was impossible to treat a patient without learning something new; it was impossible to gain fresh insight without perceiving its beneficent results" (quoted in Thomä and Kächele 1985, 1).

9. The analysis of the session dynamics, shifted content, dreams, transference, and countertransference is the way to discover unconscious desires, conflicts, and what can be called the psychological structure of the patient. An example of displaced content: a patient at the same session says about the oblong block he brought from kindergarten, then about the fear of the doctor examining his phimosis, something about the detached button—without finding any connection between the topics that seem to emerge randomly—in fact his unconscious is busy with castration anxiety; another patient talks about the wrong ways of interrogating witnesses that make people feel guilty—none of these topics concern her personally, she cannot explain where they came from, but obsessively continues to deal with them—when asked, she admits that her mother constantly made her feel guilty. An example of transference (unconscious reference to the therapist, or redirection of one's attitude towards significant figures of the past to the therapist): a patient who has just started therapy, after a long silence, says that the therapy does not give him anything, that "this method is not for him," that he expected the therapist to be more active. However, in the context of the short story about himself, it is clear that he is facing his needs of childhood—when he isolated himself in his room, he expected that one of the parents would show initiative and eventually get interested in him. He cannot show more activity in the session because he "talks" about what he experienced precisely through his inactivity. Dreams are also analyzed in the context of transference, for example: a patient dreams about a strange room as if in a hospital, meets her acquaintances there, there is also her uncle there, a doctor. She gave a baptism gift and knows that the uncle gave a more expensive one. This dream is related to her attitude to therapy, the uncle symbolizes the therapist. An example of the use of countertransference (the emotional and cognitive reactions of the therapist, that is, the emotions, sensations and fantasies the patient causes in him): feelings of discomfort, drowsiness, and a feeling of being by oneself suggest the patient's resistance, that he has cut off or suppressed some sphere of the psyche; anger at the patient may suggest that he projects a need for punishment

onto the therapist, or unconsciously desires to become a victim, wanting to prove that even therapy is evil.

10. In Kleinian terms, it is projective identification, through which one's own rage is identified as the "meanness" of the stone. Melanie Klein's theory emphasizes children's tendencies to such personifications. A child may even perceive internal states as an action of some figure, e.g., organ pain may evoke the impression in the child that it is hated (Segal 2003, 31).

11. Quotation translated from Polish by Barbara Gąstoł.

## Chapter Two

# Religion as a Neurosis, Neurosis as a Religion

## NEUROSIS AND RELIGION
## IN THE LIGHT OF PSYCHOANALYSIS

The relation between religiosity and neuroticism[1] is one of the classical issues raised by psychology of religion. Freud, in his 1907 article entitled "Obsessive Actions and Religious Practices," wrote:

I am certainly not the first person to have been struck by the resemblance between what are called obsessive actions in sufferers from nervous affections and the observances by means of which believers give expression to their piety. The term "ceremonial," which has been applied to some of these obsessive actions, is evidence of this. The resemblance, however, seems to me to be more than a superficial one, so that an insight into the origin of neurotic ceremonial may embolden us to draw inferences by analogy about the psychological processes of religious life. (Freud 1974, 117)

And hereafter:

In view of these similarities and analogies one might venture to regard obsessional neurosis as a pathological counterpart of the formation of a religion, and to describe that neurosis as an individual religiosity and religion as a universal obsessional neurosis. (Freud 1974, 126–27)

Later—in the book *Totem and Taboo*—Freud wrote about the correspondence between neurosis and two other cultural phenomena:

The neuroses exhibit on the one hand striking and far-reaching points of agreement with those great social institutions, art, religion and philosophy. But on the other hand they seem like distortions of them. It might be maintained that a

21

case of hysteria is a caricature of a work of art, that an obsessional neurosis is a caricature of a religion and that a paranoic delusion is a caricature of a philosophical system. (Freud 2004, 85)

In the quoted statements, Freud refers to the similarities between the neurotic behavior and the manifestations of individual religiosity, and to the structural analogies between neuroses and cultural products. Next to religion, he mentions art and philosophy, because both these fields are in a sense close to it. Religion is what by its essence presents human existence as one image, but art and philosophy have a similar purpose. Each of these fields is man's attempt to express, get to know, and go beyond himself. Freud's statement suggests that what we are prone to describe as "the lowest" in mental life of man (mental disorders) is related to or even "modeled" after what is "the highest" of human achievements, that is, cultural products. Is there a causal relationship here? Neuroses are to be "caricatures" of cultural products. But these products are in fact the creations of the human psyche, interestingly, often a seriously disturbed psyche, as is the case of many authors and artists. Therefore, we cannot count on simple causal relationships.

While Freud referred only to obsessional neurosis as "individual religiosity," Erich Fromm stated that every neurosis can be considered "a private form of religion," consisting in "a regression to primitive forms of religion" (Fromm 1967, 27). Fromm notes that the image of neuroses resembles the phenomena investigated by anthropology and invariably called religious:

If we scratch the surface of modern man we discover any number of individualized primitive forms of religion. Many of these are called neuroses, but one might just as well call them by their respective religious names: ancestor worship, totemism, fetishism, ritualism, the cult of cleanliness, and so on. (Fromm 1967, 29)

The understanding of the "religious" nature of these culturally patterned secular strivings is the key to the understanding of neuroses and irrational strivings. [. . .] A person whose experience is determined by "his fixation to his family," who is incapable of acting independently is in fact a worshiper of a primitive ancestor cult, and the only difference between him and millions of ancestor worshipers is that his system is private and not culturally patterned. Freud recognized the connection between religion and neurosis and explained religion as a form of neurosis, while we arrive at a conclusion that a neurosis is to be explained as a particular form of religion differing mainly by its individual, non-patterned characteristics. (Fromm 1999, 48–49)[2]

Freud perceived neurosis as the basis for explication of religion. So he must have seen it as a phenomenon with clearer contours, more basic and easier to understand. However, when we take into account his other opinion about neurosis as a religion, as well as Fromm's thesis about the need to understand the "religious nature" of neuroses, the usefulness of the reductionist position is in question. After all, both phenomena—religiousness and neuroticism—have a similar explanatory status. Reducing religion to neurosis does not explain much, because perhaps a sort of essential religiosity is the basis of neurotic functioning rather than the other way round.

But actually why neurosis? Why is this very disorder supposed to explain the phenomenon of religion? Temporal lobe epilepsy, and even more so schizophrenia could also be used here (I will come back to schizophrenia).[3] One of the reasons is probably the fact that Freud treated mainly neuroses and did not deal too much with psychoses. Of course, neuroses have aspects that allow us to think about them in the context of religion. Ceremonials of obsessive-compulsive disorder were already mentioned. Patients suffering from this disorder are also characterized by various scruples, "remorse," and in this way neuroses touch the issue of morality, so important in any religion. In neuroses, there are also manifestations of confrontation of independence and dependence, the issue of the "meaning of life," and the manifestations of irrational or magical thinking occurring in patients bring to mind the magical and ritual ways of influencing reality.

Unlike Freud, who associated any religion with obsessional neurosis, the German psychoanalyst Fritz E. Hoevels believes that only Protestantism is concurrent with this disorder, and equates Catholicism with hysterical neurosis (Hoevels 1997, 225–50).[4] He points to such attributes of Catholicism as demonstration, pomp, and even a sort of noisiness of its liturgy, in contrast to Protestantism, that is inconspicuous and modest in its expression. Catholicism is characterized by greater mobility of its followers (pilgrimages, processions, gestures made during masses) and emphasizes the community aspect of religious experiencing. Protestantism is rigid and individualistic; it concentrates on rational elements more than Catholicism, which finds expression in the recommendation of reading the Bible on one's own. It aims at a strong internalization of moral standards, which is also different in Catholicism, whose followers are more willing to trust the mercy of God. In addition, Catholicism is more strongly marked with sexual elements, clearly visible in the cult of the Virgin Mary, in kissing the feet of statues of saints, and in the narration of Catholic female mystics, who use the language of eroticism.

Based on these convergences, Hoevels considers Catholicism a mass hysteria, while Protestantism, in his view, is a mass obsessional neurosis. He further says that a given religion corresponds with a certain type of character: the hysterical character will match the Catholic doctrine and cult, while the anankastic matches the Protestant one.[5] It is, I think, not so much about the individual character as about the "social character" described by Fromm (see Fromm 2000b, 104–26), that is, the character specific to members of a given community. Fromm, on the basis of Freud's characterology and Marx's socioeconomic theory, recognized the social character as the result of the prevailing economic structure. He also considered it to be a transmitter between the economic base and the ideas promoted by society. The whole mechanism would be as follows: production relations create a kind of social interaction between people, including ways of upbringing in the family; these in turn become the cause of the emergence of certain characteristics in most members of the society; the society then accepts and develops only the ideas (statements, images) that somehow correspond to the dominant character. Religion is one of the groups of ideas and postulates supporting the aims, needs, and social ways of living of the people with the hysterical character dominant in the case of Catholicism and the anankastic one in Protestantism. Fromm also pointed to the structural convergence between feudalism and hysteria, and between capitalism and the anal character (Fromm 2000c, 204). In turn, the sociologist Max Weber addressed in his classic works the connections between the development of capitalism and Puritan ethics (Weber 1995, 88).[6] Let us add that Jung considers Protestantism to be an essentially "masculine," and Catholicism a "feminine" type of Christianity (taking into account such elements of the doctrine as the cult of the Virgin Mary in Catholicism, and the characteristics of both religions—Catholic conservatism and Protestant criticism; Jung 1995, 180 et seq.).

When we collate all the above statements, we will receive feudalism, hysteria (hysterical character), Catholicism, and "femininity" on one end, and capitalism, obsessional neurosis (anankastic character), Protestantism, and "masculinity" on the other. We notice that the elements lying on each end are saturated with one factor. But what does it mean? The authors mentioned above point to—probably not coincidental—parallels.[7] But have they known the causal mechanism of these similarities? All attempts to derive phenomena from one another turn out to be very problematic when we examine them more thoroughly.

If we compare neurosis and religion, expecting that they will relate to each other in some unambiguous way (e.g., religion will prove to be "simply a neurosis"), we will fail. If we search for their common ground only on the sociological or narrowly psychological plane we cannot be successful either. Such an attitude finds religion and neurosis as well-defined elements of reality. And yet both are something multidimensional, not fully known, just demanding understanding. In fact we can only search for common structures that concern the "symptomatology" of neurosis and religious phenomena. So it is about studying the individual, using the knowledge of both psychopathology and religion, with the focus on that individual, not on the game of the two abstractions: "religion" and "neurosis."

There is no doubt that there are connections between religion and neuroses and other mental disorders. It cannot be otherwise, because religion and psychological problems concern the basic, existential moments in human life. But we must not simply call religion a neurosis or refer to neurosis as religiousness, because in this way we would make a deeper understanding of them both impossible. We should rather start with a kind of astonishment that human beings have always sought the so-called "ways of life" as if life itself was difficult to bear. Of course, religion must be regarded as one of the "basic" ways. Also neurosis, for various reasons, is a way to deal with reality, both external and internal. It is a "way" not fully consciously chosen, not entirely wanted and not satisfactory, but shaping all life. What underlies these "ways to live" is an existential factor—something that can be called "universal maladjustment to life." It plays a part in both neurosis and religion.

## THE STRUCTURE OF NEUROTICISM

I will base the most general picture of neurosis on two pillars: the internal conflict and the remnants of the relation with caretakers. The first pillar consists of sexuality and aggressiveness, the other builds dependence. I see sexuality, aggressiveness, and dependence very extensively—as inherent elements constituting a human being.

Freud considered sexuality to be the basic area of the neurotic conflict. He presented neurosis as a result of the collision of two spheres in man: the sphere of the *ego* and the sphere of the sexual drive (Freud 1991, 26).[8] Freud's approach corresponds to the principle that applies almost to the whole organic world and is presented in the form of two "laws." The first biological law is the pursuit of an individual to preserve his life, the self-preservation instinct. The second law is the tendency to preserve the species to which the sexual drive is subordinate.[9] Without investigating which of these laws nature recognizes as prior, it must be stated that man undoubtedly combines the energies of both these instincts. They form a great fracture in his personal unity, and they are also a source of inner dynamics. Each man is torn between the tendency to focus on himself, on his own existence as an individual, and the force whose direction is not always consistent with it, the force towards the connection with another organism, towards reproduction.[10]

Neurosis is a condition in which this fracture—whether due to the weakness of the *ego*, the particular influence of the drive, or specific life events (or all of these causes)—becomes a specific problem. Neurotic symptoms are a life-sustaining compromise and serve as the bridge between the two forces mentioned above. They provide a kind of "welfare payment" that does not allow one to fully enjoy life, but at the same time helps him to survive without exposing him to the inconveniences of the labor market. A man living on a benefit will complain about the modesty of his resources, but he will also be full of fear of trying to enlarge them. The neurotic lives in a similar way. His *ego* learned the power of the second biological law, got frightened, and withdrew. However, the neurotic cannot safely close himself in the shell of his *ego*; the structure of the human psyche does not allow it. Therefore, he constantly hears the voice of the second law, but he responds to it only partially, not directly. So he is still unfulfilled, passive, halfway. This is what neurosis is: a vibrating stagnation.

The above perspective shows that neurosis is not just a "disorder." It is a reaction of the psyche to the nature of our being in the world. Its essence is the conflict between living as an "individual" and as a "part" of the collectivity. None of us is an independent monad, but no one is an undifferentiated element of the whole either. Each person struggles to reconcile the individual and supraindividual aspect. The supraindividual aspect is the umbilical cord connecting us with the whole string of generations and the laws of biological evolution. Our individuality proves to be something fragile and needs to be constantly sustained. Neurosis is a solution to the above-mentioned conflict, though not very functional. I refer to the processes related to the supraindividual aspects of the psyche as *participation*, and to the individualizing forces—as *coiling up*. I will return to these concepts.[11]

Next to the libido, another energy that builds the image of neuroses is aggression. Focusing on the conflict resulting from sexuality, Freud at first neglected this component, and later he did not explore it deeply either (Fromm 1998, 496 et seq.). However, all neurotics have problems with their own aggression, and many of the symptoms are used to channel it. The most common of these is depressiveness, which in many cases arises from an attempt to cope with aggression. By directing aggression inwards and decreasing the level of one's vitality, the neurotic prevents its expression. However, in this way, he divides himself into an accepted and excluded area more and more. That is why we can observe various, more or less severe, episodes of the dissociative nature in neurotics. I mean things that one does unwittingly, frequent oblivion, sleepwalking, not to mention involuntary movements, tics, numbness in hands or jaws, teeth grinding. These symptoms may result from attempts to cut oneself off from aggression. They appear because if we radically cut ourselves off from aggression, we also deprive ourselves of a "part" of ourselves; that is, a part of our skills, intellectual and motor capabilities, life energy. However, the fear of our own aggression can be so large that we are determined to live only partly as long as we do not have to confront it. Often the only available way to control this archaic (infantile and untamed) aggression is the mechanism of directing the drive against oneself, which manifests itself in various forms of self-destruction. The person suffers, unconsciously punishes himself, he is tense and unproductive, but at this price keeps his aggression within him. Of course, the control of aggression is a responsibility of every human being, however, the neurotic is not only afraid of its consequences, but even of its symbolic dimension, of becoming aware of it and "admitting" that it is a part of him.

The second pillar of neurosis, also consistent with Freud's statements, is the remnants of the child's dependence on caretakers. Freud presented them in detail as part of the theory about the unresolved Oedipus complex.[12] To put it more generally, we can speak of the "parental complex." It is about an affective attachment to the state of the child's dependency, about the conscious and unconscious longing for parents. Pursuant to this approach, every neurotic displays a kind of immaturity, internally remains a child and does not become fully independent. He is not really a grown-up person; deep down in his psyche, he still expects too much from others. He sees them as more powerful than himself so that they can act as parents. Thus, in a sense, he does not live among real people, but is surrounded by imaginary figures, and sees some of them as *children*, and the others as *parents*. He does not treat people as equals, as if he did not realize that all people encounter the same existential tragedy. He has the impression that he is weak and sensitive, while others are strong and life does not strike them as heavily as him. He will expect help and care from the people to whom he attributes the same powers that a child sees in its parents.

Both of the mentioned axes of neurosis remain in close relation. The neurotic cannot accept and transform the energy of the drives, because his *ego* is too weak and still dreams of support. He perceives the energy of sexuality and aggressiveness as a force that endangers his personal autonomy. On the other hand, he is afraid of this autonomy and remains, in imaginative or real terms, dependent on his parents. He is therefore "relativized" (to the relationship with the images of his parents), and at the same time "isolated" (focusing on himself and his problems). This structure causes constant tenseness. The neurotic is certainly not a person who faces his fate, taking full responsibility for himself.

## PHILOSOPHICAL DIAGNOSIS OF RELIGION

### Ludwig Feuerbach

Even before Freud, there were opinions that identified religion as a socially negative phenomenon, which is sustained by individual pathologies or triggers them. Ludwig Feuerbach was probably the first to show religion as a system that falsifies man's knowledge of himself. Feuerbach carried out a—psychological in its essence—analysis of religiosity, faith, and the idea of God. He presented the general mechanism of creation of the idea of God and the persistence of religious worship. He argued that all theology is essentially anthropology—speaking of God is a description of man. He wrote:

> Religion, at least the Christian, is the relation of man to himself, or more correctly to his own nature (i.e., his subjective nature); but a relation to it, viewed as a nature apart from his own. The divine being is nothing else than the human being, or, rather, the human nature purified, freed from the limits of the individual man, made objective—i.e., contemplated and revered as another, a distinct being. All the attributes of the divine nature are, therefore, attributes of the human nature. (Feuerbach 2008, 11–12)

Feuerbach stated that religion is the result of a kind of self-splitting of man. Believing in God along with his attributes, man implicitly expresses and reveres the qualities of his *ego*, his consciousness and mind. He divides himself into two: he keeps what is individual, conditioned, and carnal in his nature, and locates his remaining part—i.e., what goes beyond nature in him— outside himself. In this way he creates an independent being, God. What does the psychological mechanism discovered by Feuerbach consist in? Here are the examples: thinking about infinity, man thinks about the infinitude of his power of thinking; the awareness of infinity is the awareness of the infinitude of one's own awareness; the object of the religious mind is the objectified mind; the object of the religious feeling—the objectified feeling. So, for example, when the mind thinks about the absolute, the perfect or infinite object outside of itself, it only confirms its own limitlessness and perfection—it proves to itself that since it can think about something infinite, it is infinite itself. And since it cannot relate to itself directly, it watches itself in the image of God. Feuerbach wrote:

> Even the objects which are the most remote from man, *because* they are objects to him, and to the extent to which they are so, are revelations of human nature. Even the moon, the sun, the stars, call to man Γνωθισε αυτον [Know thyself]. That he sees them, and so sees them, is an evidence of his own nature. (Feuerbach 2008, 4)

So man learns only about himself, regardless of what he looks at. He learns about the entirety of what he is, about the essence of himself as a human, not through the sun or the stars, but through the idea and image of God. Feuerbach derived what is religious from the psychological transformation of the following spheres of man—the *ego*, mind, thinking, consciousness (he used these terms interchangeably) as well as the will and feelings. He described the mind as:

> the absolute subject—the subject which cannot be reduced to the object of another being, because it makes all things objects, predicates of itself,—which comprehends all things in itself, because it is itself not a thing, because it is free from all things. [. . .] The unity of the understanding is the unity of God. (Feuerbach 2008, 35)

Feuerbach's constatations about human feelings are also interesting. The philosopher notes that the all-embracing love of God, the Christian "God is love," is an expression of certainty that man's deepest desires are true and absolutely important. The feelings (the need for support, care, and protection) that overwhelm man are something divine to him, because it is impossible to transgress them. These feelings become transformed into the phantasmatic vision of God's love. It is a phantasmatic transformation of the need into fulfillment.[13] According to such a view, the greater the fulfillment the religious vision presents, the greater the need—as its source—it seems to suggest. Looking at the infinite idea of God, we can see the vastness of human needs.

Christianity and Judaism, as Feuerbach identified them, can be described as saturated with an element of narcissism. Faith in *creatio ex nihilo*, the omnipotence of God and miracles, is nothing but giving priority to the subjective over the objective world.[14] Man does not recognize here the outside world and its laws. He does not in any way limit his imagination and considers all desires as possible to be fulfilled. In the Freudian categories, we would say about the primary process and the omnipotence of thoughts. Feuerbach described religion as the "dream of waking consciousness" (Feuerbach 2008, 117). In a dream, there occurs a "reversal" of consciousness, because one perceives his emotional states and imaginations as external events and people—what he does when awake, he passively receives when asleep. Similarly with religion—there is a phantasmatic objectification of one's own internal states. This reference to the phenomenon of dream resembles the psychoanalytic approach in which dreams and dream processes are considered to be the model ones in relation to mental life.

## Karl Marx

According to Karl Marx, religion does not really present the other world, but, in a distorted way, the earth's social relations. Marx wrote:

> Religion is, in fact, the self-consciousness and self-esteem of man who has either not yet gained himself or has lost himself again. But man is no abstract being squatting outside the world. Man is the world of man, the state, society. This state, this society, produce religion, which is an inverted world-consciousness, because they are an inverted world. (Marx 1982, 131)

As one can see, Marx also regards religion as man's projection, but he sees the essence of man not in his internal world, but in social relations. For Marx, the world was an "inverted world," because it was the arena of class struggle, which, according to its aims, distorted human institutions and products of the mind. Marx pointed out that all ideologies, including religion, constitute a "false consciousness," a system of false knowledge that has no cognitive values, and is merely a correlate of the prevailing social relations. Religion arises as a kind of by-product of the defective social structure. Purely ideological contents are not the result of knowing anything, they are not any knowledge of reality. These contents *accompany* real life without describing it (this is also some form of constructivism). Regarding false social consciousness, Marx's basic observation is that mental products depend on the one who creates them. Ideologies and religion are not products of free minds, but of essentially unconscious activity. Their source is the structure of production and the network of social relations, exchange and consumption of goods. Ideologies do not say about what they say literally, but they are symptoms of the conditions of production and consumption.

These elements of Marx's theory are analogous to the psychoanalytical view, which indicates that the contents of consciousness, beliefs, and judgments are dependent on the system of drives, defenses against these drives, and internal conflicts. Each consciousness is to a certain extent a "false" consciousness, secondary rationalization or a symptom of what is really life-relevant, that is, the drive field. What the patient himself says about his "character" is always to some degree false, because this knowledge is only a part of his life process, not a reflection of it. Just as ideologies do not describe the real forces that govern social life, so man is not able to say his motivations. Although what he says about his imperatives is not accidental, it does not directly show the most important motivational forces either, it is rather their correlate ("what is the most important remains unspoken"). According to Marx, what corresponds to the drive level is the real production process, the force that really governs the individual in society.

Marx's comments on society and its products use the same perspective as the psychoanalytic approach to neurosis. Symptoms of neurosis are "compromise products," the result of the antagonistic forces that collide in the psyche. They are partly a "defense" against drives, partly a "discharge" of these drives, partly a "veil" concealing the truth about one's own life, and partly a "message" communicating the most important things. It is similar with religion. Religion, being, according to Marx, the "opium of the people," allows one to desensitize oneself to the situation of exploitation and alienation, and additionally introduces a certain degree of "abreaction." Therefore, it is a force that ensures the persistence of old social conditions. Similarly, neurosis gives a temporary satisfaction and a sense of identity, enabling the *status quo* to be maintained. And here is where the neurotic's resistance against treatment comes from. Further, although literally religion is wrong, it is a certain self-knowledge of man. Also in this respect—as being neither real nor completely pointless—it resembles a symptom. For neurosis, separating man from the truth about himself, expresses the truth at the same time. The presence of symptoms—such as anxiety, depression, obsessions, or insomnia—shows that certain things in life cannot be distorted or ignored. In turn, religious beliefs in the future happy life—if we continue to read Marx in the context of psychopathology—are like compensative fantasies of the neurotic, created in the face of the intolerable reality. For the neurotic regularly gives priority to the world of fantasy over the real life.

What is the way out of this situation? In the case of neurosis, the aim is to free the consciousness from anxieties and fixations that inhibit the individual's productivity and responsibility, and cause the necessity of living in the world of subjective symptoms, instead of the world of interpersonal relations and objective events. In the case of society and its religiously falsified consciousness, the pattern seems to be similar. Just as thanks to therapy the patient's consciousness frees itself from anxieties and perceives its place in the world more realistically, so the consciousness of all humanity will emancipate itself in the wake of revolutionary transformation. It will be nothing more than a conscious life process, in which the vivid distinction between "theory," "knowledge" or "views" and the practice of life will disappear. For this consciousness there will no longer be products of purely "idealistic" status that do not describe anything real, just as infantile fantasies cease to exist for a person who has worked through neurosis. Once society is reorganized, the conditions of production will no longer rule over man like some foreign force. Until now, it was this mysterious and uncontrollable social production process that was the main source of constraint. In this regard, it resembled the unconscious pressure which is difficult to identify with and recognize as our own, although it affects our consciousness and behavior. We sometimes treat this kind of force as an interference of something strange, a god or a demon.

## Friedrich Nietzsche

Friedrich Nietzsche's works prefigure later tendencies to see religion as a neurosis, and even directly use disease entities to refer to it. Nietzsche referred to himself as a psychologist and used the physiological and psychiatric terminology available to him to describe phenomena of culture and human behaviors. In the context of religion he spoke—using these concepts quite loosely—of neurosis, hysteria, hallucinations, neurasthenia, epilepsy, hypochondria, cyclophrenia, dissociative identity disorder, and various physiological disorders. He tried to be a naturalist, focused on the nervous system, senses, the body, vital forces, the importance of digestion, diet, and climate in the functioning of man. In human cognition he saw biological adaptation, anticipating contemporary evolutionary psychology or evolutionary epistemology. In his works, we also find similarities to many claims of psychoanalysis concerning the dynamics of human drives and the functioning of our *ego*, and his analysis of some human feelings that had been considered monolithic before is creditable.

Nietzsche passionately used psychiatric names in his attempts to understand the genesis and mechanisms of Christianity:

> We now count the greater part of the psychological apparatus with which Christianity operated as forms of hysteria and epilepsy. (Nietzsche 1968, 134)

He claimed—like Freud—that man was shaped by culture that inhibited or distorted his drives, with religion playing the leading role in this process. He wrote:

> I believe there has never been such a feeling of misery on earth, such a leaden discomfort—and at the same time the old instincts had not suddenly ceased to make their usual demands! Only it was hardly or rarely possible to humor them: as a rule they had to seek new and, as it were, subterranean gratifications. (Nietzsche 1989, 84)

This, of course, is nothing but the Freudian *Unbehagen in der Kultur*, the human discontents in culture, which does not allow direct satisfaction of the drives. Hence the indirect, "subterranean" forms of their satisfaction, which Nietzsche opposed in the name of preserving human vitality. He noted that as a result of cultural changes "hostility, cruelty, joy in persecuting, in attacking, in change, in destruction—all this turned against the possessors of such instincts: *that* is the origin of the 'bad conscience'" (Nietzsche 1989, 85). In his opinion:

> the existence on earth of an animal soul turned against itself, taking sides against itself, was something so new, profound, unheard of, enigmatic, contradictory, *and pregnant with a future* that the aspect of the earth was essentially altered. Indeed, divine spectators were needed to do justice to the spectacle that thus began. (Nietzsche 1989, 85)

Thus, the man in culture became split—Nietzsche uses the concept of *altération de la personnalité* in the context of the genesis of religion, which is a similar pattern of understanding, as in Feuerbach and Marx—there are now forces that seem to oppose him, such as the conscience or—as we could say—the *superego*. Can such a split man be strong? Nietzsche attacked Christianity because he thought that it was a manifestation of decadence, fall, the process of combating natural instincts and the vitality of the human race:

> The religious man, as the Church *wants* him, is a typical *décadent*; the moment when a religious crisis gains power over a people is always characterized by epidemics of the nerves; the "inner world" of the religious man is so like the "inner world" of the overstrained and the exhausted [. . .]. I once allowed myself to express the entire Christian repentance—*and* redemption—*training* as a methodically produced *folie circulaire.* (Nietzsche 2004b, 155–56)

Nietzsche blames religious culture for causing symptoms of bipolar disorder. He probably believes that the religious man feels angry and guilty and falls into depression at one time, and at other times, when he believes he can be saved, he falls into mania. Regarding Jesus and the kingdom of heaven, which "is not of this world," Nietzsche states:

> We recognize a condition of morbid susceptibility in the *sense of touch* which recoils in horror at every contact, every grasp of a solid object. One translates such a physiological *habitus* into its ultimate logic—as the instinctive hatred toward *every* reality, as flight into the "unintelligible," the "incomprehensible" [. . .], as being at home in a world which no kind of reality stirs any longer, an "inner world" only, a "true" world, an "eternal" world. . . . "The kingdom of God is *within you.*" (Nietzsche 2004b, 129–30)

We should rather associate Nietzsche's ideas with obsessive-compulsive disorder, which I refer to below. In it we can find aversion to "worldliness" and "temporality," which manifests itself with constant dissatisfaction with the state of reality; "hypersensitivity of the sense of touch" in the form of fear of contact with objects (explained by the fear of infection); and concentration on the internal world.

He paid much attention to compassion and pity promoted by the Christian religion, and he strongly criticized them:

> Christianity is called the religion of *pity*.—Pity stands in opposition to the tonic emotions which enhance the energy of the life-feeling: it brings about depression. One loses strength when one pities. (Nietzsche 2004b, 106)

Nietzsche claimed that compassion can be just camouflaged egoism. Someone's misfortune torments us, because it warns us about a danger to ourselves, and the failure to prevent it confronts us with a feeling of helplessness. He noticed that "benevolent revenge" can be hidden behind a pitying deed, when we help a person whom we admired or loved. This person somehow surpassed us, loving him partly deprived us of a sense of strength, which led to implicit aggressive feelings. Now that he is weak and needs our help, we can finally triumph. So Nietzsche noticed an element of ambivalence of feelings, and envy, so important in the psychoanalytical view of man.

Nietzsche opposed a healthy society and a healthy man who is active and—as he put it—says "Yes" to life, to a society and a man that is weak and reactive, governed by animosities and envy. The "ressentiment man" always looks for an external cause of his weakness; he is filled with hidden hatred, resentment, willing to get revenge. For his purposes he knows how to be "provisionally self-deprecating and humble," he does not express anything directly, and his revenge remains imaginary, poisoning his feelings (Nietzsche 1989, 38).

How does it correspond to neuroses? It seems that Nietzsche noticed an element of the dynamics of the neurotic character. Compassion can only arise in a person who does not suffer himself (as Jean-Jacques Rousseau had already noticed), for a neurotic person it may be a way to confirm his well-being and to forget about his own problems. Whereas a non-neurotic person is more likely to avoid situations in which he cannot help, but only increases his suffering from compassion, the neurotic may desire to plunge into experiencing the suffering of others. Like a woman who was interested in tragedies, such as mining catastrophes or fatal accidents, almost passionately plunging into the pain of the affected families. Of course, this could be a starting point to help others, but usually such "compassion" did not lead to anything. Could we not see camouflaged egoism here?

Undoubtedly, many neurotics represent the type criticized by Nietzsche— call it an indirect egoist. He will be constantly "apologizing for being alive," not taking into account that if something is particularly tiring for the environment, it is these continuous unproductive and essentially selfish apologies. At the same time, he will avoid realizing that this attitude is not good at all, and that his dependence can cause much more trouble to the environment than possible periodic conflicts that may result from more direct self-expression. Such people are in a camouflaged way self-centered, fearful, and incapable of constructively dedicating themselves to anything, for they have long since dedicated themselves to their suffering, that ensures peace. Nietzsche writes:

> The sick woman especially: no one can excel her in the wiles to dominate, oppress, and tyrannize. The sick woman spares nothing, living or dead; she will dig up the most deeply buried things. (Nietzsche 1989, 123)

Sick, or perhaps hypochondriac? Nietzsche indicates that, in a sense, in the "ressentiment man," the inner world is always more developed, because it suppresses many things in itself. Does this not correspond to the observation that thoughts and fantasies are overestimated in neuroses? Neurotics can create complex scenarios in which they are the heroes who save others or the bloody avengers and killers of those who displeased them. In reality, however, like the "ressentiment man" portrayed by Nietzsche, they are passive.

Nietzsche notes that culture, and Christian religion in particular, is a way to create a certain type of man—a "good" man. He is wary of such a pattern that demands:

> that mankind should do nothing evil, that it should under no circumstances do harm or desire to do harm. [. . .] This mode of thought, with which a definite type of man is bred, starts from an absurd presupposition: it takes good and evil for realities that contradict one another (not as complementary value concepts, which would be the truth), it advises taking the side of the good, it desires that the good should renounce and oppose the evil down to its ultimate roots—it therewith actually denies life, which has in all its instincts both Yes and No. (Nietzsche 1968, 192)

In a neurotic person, the attempt to divide oneself, to separate what is "bad" from what is "good" and to be only the latter grows stronger. Especially in advanced obsessive-compulsive disorder, a neurotically sensitive conscience initiates an alarm in the face of the least threat from the "bad" part. So maybe this person is a paragon of virtue? His scruples go so far that he becomes completely unproductive, and all his "moral anxiety" amounts to an idle analysis of every gesture and word. An attempt to submit to the priest, confessor, or following written rules may become an imaginary rescue. Whatever it takes to push away the unbearable responsibility. For the tormenting conscience commands to heed every thought and act, never lets anything off. Therefore, there is too much responsibility to take on. And it is not possible to take only a "part"—the obsessive person cannot evaluate such things, trivialities take on the dimension of essential things. Extreme "morality" ends with an extreme inability to bear responsibility for oneself, to decide about oneself and, finally, with an inability to have healthy relationships with other people. What does Nietzsche say about it? He states something that probably many people find difficult to accept:

> For every strong and natural species of man, love and hate, gratitude and revenge, good nature and anger, affirmative acts and negative acts, belong together. One is good on condition one also knows how to be evil; one is evil because otherwise one would not understand how to be good. (Nietzsche 1968, 191)

Not only religion is the way to be "good." A disease can also become a way of one's own "sanctification." Nietzsche says that "one is good in a sickly manner when one is sick" (Nietzsche 1968, 134). We can indeed say that in neuroses and some personality disorders one is often convinced of "being good" due to being sick. A person suffering from neurosis is "good" because he is a "victim." He then can show his suffering to the others and expect help from them, which Freud called the secondary gains of illness. Having adopted the attitude of a martyr, he can feel morally better this way, for he purportedly bears the suffering that is unknown to others. But is not such an attitude a kind of deception? If we just took the liberty of being joyful and healthy, we would have to become responsible for ourselves and thus directly encounter the tragedy of life and perhaps the feeling of loneliness.

Neurotics want care and compassion, and therefore they may be afraid that someone will see their hidden anger, aggression, greed or egoism. In general, these elements can be described as "individualizing," they indicate that one is a separate being. And this means that contacts with others will never take the form of a conflict-free flow. Aggression separates from people, but also requires face-to-face confrontation. If one acknowledges the aggression of others he also acknowledges their autonomy, existence independent of his own needs and desires. Let us illustrate this with an example: during a group therapy, a patient takes another one's hand, after she told about some difficult experience. This action leads to superficial harmony and reassurance. However, it prevents further verbalization and confrontation of differences, it blocks mutual cognition. It also prevents seeing oneself as a separate individual. Perhaps it indicates lack of strength to recognize and accept the other in his otherness.

The neurotic becomes "good" because he has blocked the expression of sexuality or aggressiveness. These elements can be so repressed that a person disposes of all his assertiveness and productivity. Sexuality and aggressiveness, as too threatening to the *ego*, become banned, considered "evil." These energetically basic aspects of life are, anyway, predestined to be avoided, rejected, and negatively evaluated, because they constantly threaten social coexistence and the existence of the individual. Unrestrained sexuality can become a source of conflicts with the environment and the cause of one's doom. The expression of one's own aggression can expose one to the aggression of others. The drives are a challenge for every human being, nobody is born with their full understanding or the ability to control them, and society offers very few constructive methods of mastering them. What underlies their negative evaluation is fear. In this situation, a man who suppresses the expression of these drives, begins to convince himself and everyone else that his current attitude proves his "goodness" and disgust for "evil." Nietzsche recognized reaction formations—as psychoanalysis would call them—and manifestations of the hidden activity of the drive, the sexual one for example, also in phenomena that were far from it, such as ecstasies of mystics. Religious fervor manifests itself in many cases as "the disguise of a girl's or youth's puberty" or as "the hysteria of an old maid" (Nietzsche 2017, 53). Nietzsche particularly disliked priests in whom he saw lack of "psychological cleanliness" similarly to "hysterical females" and "rickets-laden children" who never look in the eye and tend to falsify and deceive (Nietzsche 2004b, 157).

To what extent is this need for "goodness" at the price of symptoms, self-deception, and nonproductivity stimulated by religious culture, and how much is it determined by the factor of life in community in general, or by intrapsychological conditions? Irrespective of the possible causative factors, the structure of neurotic behavior can be compared to bigotry. Religion is similar to neurosis in that it can make one believe in the existence of a life niche, allowing him to easily become "better than others." Some people who live there, believe that perfection can be achieved by adopting a certain way of being, behaving in a given way, and sticking to a certain set of ideas. Nietzsche writes:

> These little herd-animal virtues do not by any means lead to "eternal life": to put them on show in this way, and oneself with them, may be very clever but to him who keeps his eyes open even here, it remains in spite of all the most ludicrous of all plays. One does not by any means deserve a privileged position on earth and in heaven by attaining perfection as a little, good-natured sheep; one remains at best a little, good-natured, absurd sheep with horns—provided one does not burst with vanity—as the court chaplains do—or provoke scandal by posing as a judge. (Nietzsche 1968, 119)

Manipulations that are supposed to make us "good" can concentrate on things as trivial as the way we express ourselves, the tone of voice we adopt, the melody of our speech. For example, priests use a characteristically modulated voice, but this area of expression is controlled by many other people as well. It is difficult to characterize sounds in the written word, but we can say that the goal of such modifications is to avoid the phonic components of speech that are associated with the expression of drives. The voice becomes monotonous, ingratiating, unnaturally elevated or specifically childish. There are many similar ways to superficially transform one's identity (artificial and endless kindness and warmth, excessive self-control, false fullness of rationality, excessive tolerance and openness). Is it the Christian culture that promoted the vision of man nobody will ever reach without suppression, self-deception, and pose? Probably not only it.

It seems that it is difficult for neurotics to accept that they could differ from the image imposed by the cultural stereotype. They are not mature enough to be able to bear their own "evil." Fitting the social model is very important for them. And yet the Christian religion itself recommends that we transgress our social conditions, see them as relative and not meaningful ("Blessed are ye when men shall reproach you, and persecute you, and say all manner of evil against you falsely, for my sake. Rejoice, and be exceeding glad: for great is your reward in heaven: for so persecuted they the prophets that were before you," Matthew 5:11–12; "For what shall a man be profited, if he shall gain the whole world, and forfeit his life? or what shall a man give in exchange for his life?," Matthew 16:26). However, few can really follow this path.

Nietzsche points to a specific escape from one's own *ego* and plunging into the opinions that others have about us, which is probably a manifestation of our "herd" instincts:

> Whatever they may think and say about their "egoism," the great majority nonetheless do nothing for the phantom of their ego which has formed itself in the heads of those around them and has been communicated to them;—as a consequence they all of them dwell in a fog of impersonal, semi-personal opinions, and arbitrary, as it were poetical evaluations, the one for ever in the heads of others: a strange world of phantasms—which at the same time knows how to put on so sober an appearance! (Nietzsche 2003, 106)

A particular type of withdrawal is found in neurotic women, who can be described as "women-who-have-never-cared-about-themselves." That is how they describe themselves, "I never cared about myself," "I always did everything for my family," "I could not take care of myself," and sometimes they add, "And now I broke down." This attitude, like any psychological attitude, is complicated and difficult to unequivocally assess. The described women are indeed victims of their sacrifices, but at the same time they are prisoners of their egoism. In an ingenious way, they gave up their responsibility for themselves. Somehow they outstretched their person in a network of relationships and obligations, which meant that they did not have to confront face-to-face with their partners, children, or other people. They denied that they had egoistic needs and built their identity around their great "goodness." They sacrificed their true *ego* in favor of the image of their *ego* present in the "heads of those around them."

Christianity and Buddhism, in Nietzsche's opinion, are nihilistic religions. The difference is that Buddhism, being a religion of the natural end of civilization, encourages us to get rid of our vital forces in a gentle and unintrusive way, and Christianity demands a fight and an active suppression of the energy of life and drives. Nietzsche approaches the problem of religion "physiologically" and states that in advanced culture, such as Hindu, there is—whatever he means exactly—"a refined capacity for pain," and "over-intellectuality" as a result of "too great preoccupation with concepts and logical procedures" and for these reasons "a state of *depression* has arisen: against this Buddha takes hygienic measures" (Nietzsche 2004b, 118). So Buddhism is a kind of healing system in nihilistic reality, based on softening affects, diet, promoting calming images. The author sees that man depressively suffers in both religions, but Christianity seems to have sadistic elements, because it is based on "an overwhelming desire for painmaking, for the release of inner tension in hostile actions and conceptions" (Nietzsche 2004b, 120). Nietzsche, however, is a thinker who adopted a dynamic way of explaining—he sees processes and the clash of contradictory forces. Christianity not only destroys but is also a salvation—its "ascetic ideal is an artifice for the *preservation* of life" (Nietzsche 1989, 120). However, this ideal of sacrifice and suppression, "this hatred of the human, and even more of the animal, and more still of the material," this fear of life and happiness, escape from change, death and desire, shows a certain direction and sense (Nietzsche 1989, 162–63). Human suffering has been interpreted in terms of guilt. Thus, however, as Nietzsche states, "the door was closed to any kind of suicidal nihilism" and "man was *saved* thereby, he possessed a meaning, he was henceforth no longer like a leaf in the wind, a plaything of nonsense," "he could now *will* something" (Nietzsche 1989, 162).

## Does This Explain Religion?

The authors mentioned above fought against religion for the sake of restoring man's dignity, vitality, and creative potential. They wanted to show him the way to adulthood and responsibility for himself and the world. They postulated that people, instead of hypochondriacally complaining about temporality and waiting for the Kingdom of God, should undertake a heroic effort to improve their individual and social lives. They did not want to recognize religion, because they claimed it made man delude himself that he would achieve something of value, and he in fact remained under the influence of a phantasm. In this regard, they took a stance that was identical to that of Freud, who underlined the necessity of an "education to reality" (Freud 1961b, 49), recommending to reject the infantile and false pillars of our fate (such as the image of God) and confront reality. All the three authors used concepts that described the psychological mechanisms of negating reality and producing substitutive visions, which is close to the psychoanalytical approach. They wrote about consciousness and its falsifications. Did Feuerbach, Marx, and Nietzsche teach us something about the psychology of religion?

Feuerbach's philosophy does not explain all religious phenomena, focusing primarily on the theological vision of God. It does not explain mystical states, shamanism, or even the cult of the Mother of God. According to Feuerbach, man tends to objectify his inner states, and that is why we live in the world of our own projections. It is difficult for us to perceive ourselves, and we must analyze our products and ideas in order to get to know ourselves. The image of God tells us about ourselves. The question is, Can we withdraw all our projections and see ourselves only in ourselves? Or does a part of ourselves always have to remain "outside"? Marx's claims are not unfounded—the content and form of religious worship are sociologically conditioned; they depend on the material basis of life and the structure of social relations.[15] Man's alienation, his enslavement by the conditions of production and exchange of goods, results in the continuing of faith in the existence of something supernatural. They, like God, rule over people. When people consciously plan the production process and use the fruits of their own work, then happiness, which until now was to be obtained through the illusory vision of paradise, will now be achievable on earth. In the psyche of a free man, the libidinal cathexis will be withdrawn from the religious fantasies and they—to use the language of psychoanalysis—deprived of energy, will disappear completely. To refer to Freud's words: where *It* was, there shall *I* become.[16]

However, can the quality of human existence change so much that his psyche transforms completely? Only then all the forces supporting the existence of religion would really be eliminated. The secularization of rich societies seems to confirm that the quality of life matters here. Wealth really draws people away from institutional religions. However, all this is happening in the capitalist countries, so where human alienation has not been eliminated, thereby no radical changes in the psyche have occurred. Even if fewer people are traditionally religious, magical, wishful, conspiratorial and fantastic thinking flourishes.

Marx thought that man and his needs would change completely in the society of the future—all human problems would be absorbed by the community and resolved. In the communist society, even the problem of death was to lose its meaning—a person united with others would not feel the fear of it anymore. Such a psychological process does exist—emotional bonding with others means that we are less anxious about ourselves, while lonely neurotics are always hypochondriacal, showing intense concerns about their lives. On the other hand, social exclusion is one of the most painful situations for man, which he may fear more than death. So would a "proper" society eliminate all our fears and hesitations?

Marx, in fact, presented a vision similar to that of all religions—the ultimate peace of being and harmony. He believed that the transformation of man can happen on earth, through the transformation of the social structure and the end of the class struggle. The idea is certainly too optimistic, for it assumes that a radical and ultimate transformation of man and humanity will take place without the transformation of the cosmos, the Earth, human physiology, and many other things. Unless we believe Leon Trotsky, who argued that the new man would be able to "harmonize himself" and, moreover, he would try:

> to master first the semiconscious and then the subconscious processes in his own organism, such as breathing, the circulation of the blood, digestion, reproduction, and, within necessary limits, he will try to subordinate them to the control of reason and will. [. . .] Emancipated man will want to attain a greater equilibrium in the work of his organs and a more proportional developing and wearing out of his tissues, in order to reduce the fear of death to a rational reaction of the organism toward danger. There can be no doubt that man's extreme anatomical and physiological disharmony, that is, the extreme disproportion in the growth and wearing out of organs and tissues, give the life instinct the form of a pinched, morbid, and hysterical fear of death, which darkens reason, and which feeds the stupid and humiliating, and which feeds the stupid and humiliating fantasies about life after death. Man will make it his purpose to master his own feelings, to raise his instincts to the heights of consciousness, to make them transparent, to extend the wires of his will into hidden recesses, and thereby to raise himself to a new plane, to create a higher social biologic type, or, if you please, a superman. (Trotsky 2005, 206–207)

The first step would probably be to heal one's own neuroses. However, if someone thinks that working through neurosis can free him from all fears and uncertainties, he will be disappointed. It is true that he will dispose of inadequate neurotic anxieties, but he will at the same time expose himself to the universal existential fears.

Despite many accurate, deep, psychological or historiosophic insights, Nietzsche's literature seems to be an attempt to cope with his own problems. I see the voice of a psychotic, probably a genius, but lonely and plunged into grandiose fantasies, switching from mania to depression.[17] Nietzsche presents himself as a completely unique person, as a "psychologist without equal," a prophet, a person with an unusual ability to feel. And all this in a radical context of "never," "none," "only" ("for I come from heights that no bird ever reached in its flight, I know abysses into which no foot ever strayed;" Nietzsche 1989, 263).

Nietzsche's dislike, even hatred, of his mother and sister is characteristic. He writes:

> I am a pure-blooded Polish nobleman without a single drop of bad blood, certainly not German blood. When I look for my diametric opposite, an immeasurably shabby instinct, I always think of my mother and sister,—it would blaspheme my divinity to think that I am related to this sort of *canaille*. (Nietzsche 2005, 77)

Nietzsche describes his father, who died at the age of thirty-six, as a frail, kind, and morbid man. He says that he, too, felt the weakest at the same age. The hatred of the mother and the kind of longing for the father are quite typical of psychoses. It is difficult for the psychotic to tolerate his mother, as will be discussed in this book. In all his works, Nietzsche criticizes and rejects the Germans in the same way as he criticizes and rejects his mother, building his own identity. He seeks for a strong and active man he would probably want to see in his father and to become himself. The strong father would protect him from his terrible mother, just as "decadent" as his contemporary culture and morality.

In my opinion, the rather naive reference to physiology, especially the "gastric system," digestion and diet, is also of the psychotic character. We can observe something similar in some people in psychosis when they smoothly pass from symbolic or psychological to physiological statements. For example, such a person may immediately move from the question of "good taste" to the issue of nutrition (Kleinian psychoanalysts in a similar context speak of "symbolic equation;" Segal 2006, 84). Nietzsche believed that his hands revealed his inner spirit, he also attributed great importance to the shape of his ears, which he said were the ears "for the unheard" (Frenzel 1994, 111). He was said to be sensitive to "every cloud that appears in the sky" and felt when the air was "more full of electricity" (Hollingdale 2001, 127, 129). Nietzsche treated all this quite seriously. These are manifestations of "psychotic psychosomatics"—characteristic of many psychotics, and bizarre for a listener, combining psychological and physical feelings, body and spirit.

Nietzsche—an eulogist of the "proud soul," asserting that compassion is a deception and evil, because it makes not only one weak but two, one day, sobbing out of compassion, hugged a horse beaten by a cabman. Then the period of his manifest psychosis started. He began to write letters to the courts of Europe, announced he would arrive as Dionysius and the Crucified one, he regarded the wife of his former friend, Richard Wagner, as his own and called her Ariadne. He was admitted to a psychiatric clinic, and eventually his mother and sister attended to him. The eternal traveler did not want to leave his house anymore, the critic of religion became more and more absorbed in a "religious mood" (Hollingdale 2001, 246).

The career of Nietzsche's life shows the importance of religion in the mind of a psychotic, which I refer to later in this book. As a young man, Nietzsche was very religious, then he fought against religion, to return to religious themes later. In the meantime, he tried to be the greatest psychologist, a person wiser than all physicians, a prophet who would "shoot the history of mankind into two halves" (Hollingdale 2001, 197). At the end, he identified himself with divine figures who, in his works, were to be only metaphors and personifications of ideas.

## OBSESSIVE-COMPULSIVE DISORDER—THE DENIAL OF TEMPORALITY

### Obsessive-Compulsive Disorder—"Religious" Neurosis

Obsessive-compulsive disorder (obsessional neurosis) is a mental problem that is, for a reason, associated with religiosity. In regard to the observed behaviors, it consists in performing specific, monotonous, and impractical activities by the patient. Subjectively, its essence is recurrent thoughts or impulses and anxiety. The severe form of obsessive-compulsive disorder involves a distinctive change in personality. Man not only *has symptoms*, but also takes a specific approach to almost all spheres of life, especially those related to relationships, family, love and sexuality, plans, and the future.

When we speak of the "neurotic ritual," we mean a combination of activities that are performed with a significant frequency and in a relatively fixed manner. Compulsory activities are by no means pleasant for the sick person, he performs them out of necessity and sometimes tries to oppose the impulse that motivates him, but failing to perform the activities would result in a hundred times greater discomfort. As Freud writes, the ceremonial becomes a kind of "sacred act" (Freud 1974, 118), and abandoning it invariably leads to tension and anxiety.

For hundreds of years obsessions have been associated with religious contents. John Bunyan, a seventeenth-century English writer and Puritan preacher, the author of *The Pilgrim's Progress*, could not resist the obsessive thought to "sell Christ" (Rosenhan and Seligman 1994, 277). "Sell him, sell him, sell him" appeared in his mind "as fast as a man could speak." The answer was the words to negate, we would say "undo," the above: "No, no, not for thousands, thousands, thousands," repeated at least twenty times in a row (Bunyan 1845, 32).

Even if we accepted the thesis that religious obsessions are less common nowadays than in earlier times (Rosenhan and Seligman 1994, 277–78), we would have to say anyway that religious elements are still observed, not infrequently. Thoughts or words, considered blasphemous by the patient himself, are frequent and may co-exist alongside other symptoms of neurosis. The sphere of *sacrum*, as the area of something absolute, maximally sacred or cursed, remains an attractor focusing extreme emotions that occur in this disorder.

## Splitting in Obsessive-Compulsive Disorder

In my therapeutic practice, it happened several times that people with obsessive-compulsive disorder described their state as similar to demonic possession.[18] Sometimes, due to the blasphemous nature of their obsessive thoughts, they were ready to accept the possibility that the thoughts were sent by the devil himself.

Let us look at a similar phenomenon, which, however, remains within the range of normality—at involuntary blasphemous thoughts that occur in adolescents at the age of puberty. These thoughts appear particularly often and obsessively when in the church and include sexual and obscene content. The mechanism of these obsessions results from awakening of sexual impulses during puberty and from the repressive nature of religious culture. A young man faces a situation in which what he feels is basically different from the preferred pattern. The values manifested by the environment, which earlier (in the latency period)[19] seemed to fit his internal needs, now turn out to be in conflict with them. In his own eyes, the adolescent becomes marked and socially unfit, and experiences culture as a constricting corset. He dreams of disposing of it, and at the same time is terrified of what could happen then. Experiencing the exalted atmosphere of the church can bring the most obscene and vulgar thoughts. The more intensively the ban is experienced, the stronger the tendency to break it. Obsessive fantasies about sexuality or nudity of the saints, being the voice of the drive sphere, are supposed to negate their repressive character.

The person, overcome by obsessions, feels the stratification of his psyche in a particularly strong way. What happens to him can often be compared to the battle of Dr. Jekyll and Mr. Hyde in the common body. He may, more or less clearly, see and feel within himself the existence of "someone else." This "other being" constantly endangers what the person identifies with. The patient wants to be one, a person adapted to the outside and peaceful inside, but the "other one" constantly ruins his plans.

This fear of oneself is not completely groundless. For there are wild and untamed impulses under the mask of peace and control. In the development of the person with obsessions, a long-lasting process of isolating and suppressing a significant part of himself must have taken place. Certain impulses were isolated throughout his life, and his identity was built as their antithesis. This resulted in the formation of two separate poles—the "good" and socially adapted, and the crazy and aggressive one. The person suffering from obsessions may perceive the latter pole of himself as a demon.

In obsessive-compulsive disorder, the person wants to establish clear boundaries between himself and the world as well as the ones in himself, at the same time constantly feeling that these boundaries are missing. For example, a man may have the compulsion to share his thoughts with his partner regarding other women. He will torment her telling her that he looked at a woman, he thought something, etc. He will also torment himself thinking what else he should tell her. It is difficult for him to keep these matters "to himself," as if he had no "room" for them inside, as if he did not have any boundaries within which he could close them. The boundary problem may also apply to the physical space. The obsessive person may, for example, have the impression that someone touched and dirtied him, although the distance from that person was in fact considerable. However, the obsessive neurotic is not sure if it was actually half a meter or if, in some strange way, there was a contact.

The problem of boundaries is related to splitting we address here. The idealized part of the *self* tends to *coil up*, the rest is in *participation*. For this reason, many experiences "do not fall within the ambit" of the part of the man with whom he wants to identify himself (the idealized *self*). This second, rejected part, is thus "thrown out" to the outside world. For the obsessive person it "blends" with externality, which makes externality cease to be the pure *not-me*, he can no longer distance himself from it, which makes him so sensitive to the environment (dirt, feces, bacteria, and other threats). Through his quest for isolation, the obsessive person becomes, to an absurd extent, open to what comes from the outside. Therefore, the distance may cease to matter to him and he might become afraid of a hot stove standing two meters away. The normal causal relationships also disappear and the neurotic has the impression that he will cause an airplane crash with his thoughts. Also, because of the described lack of boundaries, he reacts so strongly to any disturbances in the environment (from symmetry, order, and noise outside the window to the political situation of the country).

## The Fear of Existential Freedom

Compulsive rituals can vary, but they can be grouped into a few categories. One of them is excessive cleanliness, which may consist in constant washing oneself, caring for freshness of bedding and clothing, isolating "dirty" items from those that are to remain absolutely clean. Compulsive checking is another group. The patient checks for several dozen times whether he closed the door, turned off the gas. Making the same gesture, he repeatedly "checks" whether he accidentally hit his genitals. The third group is care for order and symmetry as well as activities such as avoiding stepping on the joints of pavement tiles and compulsive counting (of activities or objects). The fourth one includes activities related to religious objects and content, such as compulsively making the sign of the cross, kissing statues or pictures, or multiple utterings of certain phrases.

What is the function of each of these activities? They are to protect against threatening thoughts and impulses. These compulsive impulses, often not fully aware, concern strictly defined areas. Generally speaking, sexuality and aggressiveness, including self-destruction. Thus, a mother may experience obsessive fear of her child's death, someone else will not be able to resist blasphemous thoughts, another woman will fight the impulse ordering her to throw her child out of the window or the tendency to fall under a speeding car.

Note that compulsive routines converge in a point that may be determined by concepts such as perfection, potency, security. Whereas, impulses are dangerous and aggressive factors. That is why obsessive-compulsive disorder is an internal struggle. The man overwhelmed with obsessions and compulsions seeks extraordinary safety for himself, while the other side of his psyche constantly offers visions of danger. Why is he worried that he will not turn off the gas or leave something on the bus? Because he has a feeling that he could start acting to the detriment of himself.

Where does this idea come from? What scares the neurotic is existential freedom. It is this kind of freedom that deprives of the sense of security, telling that "everything is possible," that man has no self-protection against himself (nothing and no one will stop the suicide's hand). Feeling that at any moment he can become a threat to himself (both through direct attack on himself and through the explosion of aggression against the environment), the patient nips spontaneous impulses in the bud, becoming overly cautious. Trying to reject all risks from himself, he closes himself in the shell of ritual activities, and becomes inflexible inside.

## Logos and Chaos—the Ceremonial and Variability of Things

Obsessive-compulsive disorder is a rejection of the passage of time and the variability of life, it is an extreme intolerance of the theologically understood "temporality" and the imperfection of the world. This intolerance is built primarily on the basis of internal splitting, which I mentioned above. The affirmed area is isolated from what is imperfect, dependent, and impulsive. This is to ensure peace, safety, and self-appeasement. The person with obsessive-compulsive disorder wants to avoid contact with reality, preferring fantasies and his or her own artificial sense of security.

The *ego* of the obsessive-compulsive patient sticks to the sphere of meanings in a particularly strong way, and avoids the "thing in itself"[20] to a large extent. The patient does not tolerate what is vague and illogical, in general: the unsymbolizable. He wants to escape from emotions, coincidence, uncertainty, and the opacity of interpersonal relations. He chooses the symbolic world of the mind, the area of fantasy and purely mental connections (controlling one's thoughts, undoing, etc.). This pursuit is so strong as if the man wanted to *identify* with what is logical and mental, he even wants to be the *logos*, to exist as the *nous*. He prefers mental representations to the real life process, because the conceptual, symbolic, or imaginary is permanent, it is beyond time.

The ceremonial is to replace the evolutionary course of events with the cyclical time, to somehow cheat time, closing its course into a loop. This is to allow one to live next to the world of change. The neurotic, of course, senses that time passes and each day brings a new situation, but is afraid of changes more than others. Although deep changes are dangerous for all of us (the whole body tries, after all, to keep homeostasis, that is, the internal environment with relatively limited variability), the man with obsessive-compulsive disorder fears changes in a particularly strong way. His ability to tolerate changes has never been sufficiently developed. And he built something that he perceives as permanent at the expense of experiencing neurotic symptoms.

The process of the passage of time is a threat to him because, among other things, it is associated with the anticipation of punishment and defeat born from the unconscious sense of guilt. The ritual is to make "tomorrow not come," to make everything remain the same (extreme attachment to order and monotony is a kind of negation of entropy). However, from the inside (or rather from the "inside-outside") the opposite presses, and wants to disrupt this attitude.

Someone may fear infection, for example. In order to avoid it, he makes his endless toilet. However, this remedy begins to go beyond the realm of the body, as if the washing was to wash the soul too. Washing is disposing of dirt, but in the case of washing that repeats several or dozens of times in an hour, there can be no real dirt. Nevertheless, the person overwhelmed with the compulsion feels the dirt of his hands. The belief that his hands are dirty is a projection of his internal state. It is primarily repressed rage, which is perceived as something "contagious," something that almost accumulates on the surface of the body, threatening both the environment and the sick. Undoubtedly, the sense of guilt matters here. However, the man is not clearly aware of it, because repression and the ceremonial protect him from realizing it.[21]

A young woman, a nurse, was constantly afraid that she might be infected with HCV and infect others, she was also afraid that her alleged negligence at work would lead some of the patients to death. These obsessive fears were close to delusions, because the woman could not accept rational arguments. Psychotherapy showed that the main reason for the formation of these symptoms was the patient's ambivalent relationship with her mother. The woman lived with her and she was dependent on her, experiencing it as a burden and being afraid of independence at the same time. In addition, the mother—who raised her daughter so that she would be dependent—implied that her daughter's attitude did not suit her. At the same time, she claimed that she would do everything best and did not want to share even the simplest housework activities with the daughter. The patient had never experienced the rebellion stage, and she was now torn between the need for maternal care and anger about her attitude. On the direct, conscious level, she could not express her aggression in any way, or even confront it. However, this repressed aggression towards the mother caused a sense of guilt, which took the form of fear of punishment (infection). This aggression was also directed at others, which manifested itself as the fear of harming someone (by failing to fulfill her duties or infecting someone). In this way, the idea of infection served as neutralization of guilt and partial expression of aggression.

Obsessive-compulsive disorder involves the process of shifting, which means that the affective investment is transferred to the compulsive activity from another object or activity. The act then becomes similar to religious ceremonies, because it is considered to be necessary, and at the same time it has no rational grounds. However, it is always—like any other symptom of neurosis—a compromise product. It blocks impulses and needs and at the same time it meets them to some extent. The ritual always conceals something weighty. The ceremonial hides it on the one hand, and on the other it points to it and is a form of its indirect expression. An obsessive thought both "commands" to deal with the weighty matter, and isolates the mind from its essence. In this situation, obsession stops the man halfway. It is an attempt to find one's own place in life, without becoming aware, making decisions and taking responsibility for oneself.

We are all subject to transience, which for each of us is an ongoing, unresolved problem. The matter of transience, alongside love, is perhaps the basic theme that drives culture (painting, poetry, prose, theater, and film). There are probably no other more human-specific questions than these: "Will a part of me survive?," "Is there anything permanent in this world?" Neurosis also "addresses" these questions. The patient, through obsessions and compulsions, tries to establish some stability in the constant flow of life. He feels more clearly than others that there is nothing permanent, because his *ego* is exposed to the influence of particularly impulsive and primordial emotions. The fear of splitting the *ego*, that is, the fear of madness, underlies the multiplied sense of instability of life in people with obsessive-compulsive disorder. The accurate performance of the ritual is to prevent the suppressed pursuits from surfacing, which could threaten the integrity of the *ego*.

## As the World Attacks—Clinical Case Study

Andrew,[22] a middle-aged man, has struggled with obsessive-compulsive symptoms since he was a child. In the beginning he involuntarily imagined that the sculptures he saw in the church were naked. This particularly applied to the statue of the Virgin Mary. He also remembered he was severely tense between confession and receiving the Holy Eucharist. It seemed to him that something "attacked" him, telling him to "defile" himself. In order to resist the tiring thoughts, he shook his head, then he experienced "emptiness" in the head and could somehow make it to receive the sacrament. After communion, he had a feeling of calm and bliss.

Andrew's biography includes the element, which Freud associated with the etiology of obsessional neurosis—premature sexual activity (Freud 1996, 31). The patient, when he was eight years old, experienced a series of sexual intercourses with a six years older girl. He found them very pleasant, but soon the girl started using him for various purposes, blackmailing him that if he did not obey her, she would stop having sex with him. After a short time they became hostile to each other. Since then, he was constantly thinking about sex, and his symptoms began to form soon after these events. The first was to compulsively touch his heels while walking, in turns left and right.

The sexual relationship in his childhood prematurely awakened strong sexual needs that could not be satisfied. This situation gave birth to two phenomena that would affect Andrew's later life: growing frustration and withdrawal into the world of fantasy (Andrew used sexual fantasies and accompanying masturbation to cope with insomnia). But what is the core of the trauma here, since the sexual experience was perceived as pleasant and desirable? Well, what negatively determined Andrew's later life was the fact that his immature psyche came into contact with sexual intercourse, which is by nature incomprehensible, that is, the *real*.

Andrew, on the one hand, began to desire sexual intercourse, and on the other, he was horrified by its mystery and hard "reality." That is why he basically began to desire not the real intercourse, but the intercourse of his fantasies. Thus, not only the lack of a partner, but also the unconscious fear of reality, made him withdraw into the imaginary world of sexual satisfaction and gradually retreat from the real world.

Andrew was more and more split into the realm of the imaginary, ideal, and potentially satisfied *ego*, and the area of aggression caused by frustration, which he wanted to keep away from his consciousness. He experienced the latter sphere as an immense reservoir of energy that he could not cope with, and that "attacked" him (he described it as a black eagle lunging at him). This energy manifested itself in continuous muscle tension and tics. When he sat or stood, he looked as if he had to hold a wild animal under his skin. Tension and tics intensified when he raised a difficult issue or when something unpleasant came to his mind. He then clenched his hands on the armrests of the chair, struggling to calm down, and muttered with gritted teeth: "fuck . . . sorry . . . sorry . . . God . . . calm . . . calm. . . ."

Andrew did not identify himself with the untamed sphere of the *self*, wanting to block it and reject from the consciousness. He saw himself as a sensitive person, capable of "the highest feelings," with a particularly refined taste for music. He often sat in an armchair and fell into musical ecstasy—he felt then that he was "great." However, the more he identified with the idealized *ego*, the more unbearable the randomness and imperfection of the world became. A noise outside the window, a small defect in the apartment, or an uninvited visit of the neighbor was enough for him to start to furiously curse, tremble, and perform his compulsive rituals with an increased intensity. In order to become calm again, he got isolated even more, trying even harder to cut himself off from the chaotic and unbridled part of him and of the world.

Andrew remembered that in his youth, when he was to go to a party, where he expected music, alcohol, and girls, so this what he enjoyed, he got "mad" and "paced the floor," unable to leave. As if something blocked his joy and did not let him be happy. Similarly, for example, when he planned to eat something good. Good food extremely pleased him, but as soon as tasting was possible, compulsions started as well—he could not stop washing his hands, checking, etc.

What do these opposing forces mean? We can understand them as a compensating voice of his unconscious, which says: "Your joy is unrealistic, you want to experience angelic moments without blemish, come to your senses, it is impossible." Andrew was only able to enjoy fantasies, not reality. If a situation seemed to him particularly pleasant, close to his dreams, he not only craved for it, but unconsciously began to immensely fear it. For the situation that is *closest* to the fantasy is also the biggest threat to it.

When Andrew was to meet a woman, the moment of waiting, the play of the imagination, was the most important moment for him. When he had sex, he never thought about his partner, but imagined another woman he had not slept with before. If he happened to think about the partner, he could not breathe normally and lost interest in sex. He often preferred to just watch women than sleep with them—the woman could be old and unattractive, but by the fact that she was an image, she became more attractive. He was attracted to and became aroused by idealized images, but when he came into contact with a real woman, he had to make sure that she differed from the ideal. In this way, he avoided the combination of reality and dreams, and thus protected the most exciting, that is, his world of fantasy.

In order to keep the untamed part of himself away and reject what is incomprehensible in the world, Andrew controlled the logic and clarity of his statements and carefully chose the words he used. He almost worshiped some words, he liked to utter them. He did not speak the language only to express reality and make contacts with people, but also to maintain his identification with the mind. Although he described himself as a person primarily driven by emotions—which in a sense was true—he could only bear what was named, rational and semantically transparent.

As opposed to his linguistic accuracy, he was unable to talk about many aspects of his life, such as some situations in the past and relations with some people. When he was about to say something about his former mother-in-law, the neighbor or the relationship with his brother, he got uncontrollable tics, grabbed the armrest, and had to change the topic to calm down. He could hardly say anything about these people; he could only utter insults against them. Also, he could not comfortably analyze the situations associated with these people. It did not result from the mere anger that may be elicited by the need to remember someone one dislikes or considers an enemy. In their presence he came into contact with reality, which he tried to avoid. These people and their behavior could not be symbolically tamed in a simple way. He could not "treat them as part of the background" and just stay in his own world. Through their selfishness, brutality, directness, or even simple emotionality, these people invaded his mental, idealized world, sowing chaos. The *real* reached him in the form of the vulgar neighbor or in the person of the brother he hated.

Everyone can experience a similar situation, where they may feel misunderstood or not understand the other person, so the contact may be like meeting a stranger. However, we usually deal with the situations that involve lack of agreement and common meanings. Andrew did not have this skill. He could not delve into something that was beyond his usual view, or tolerate it. The sphere of his mind was organized so rigidly that he was incapable of accepting something that did not fit into his cognitive patterns and fantasies. We must remember that this is not about "simple" mental inflexibility and the resulting limitation of creative intelligence, but about a deeper cause. The cause was Andrew's identification with the sphere of clearly defined meanings.

Andrew clung to certain reflections, ideas, and imaginations for fear of deconstructing himself as a self-determining subject. We all know that breaking the image of ourselves, someone's contrary allusion, or opinion on ourselves can trigger a strong and very unpleasant reaction, bordering on a sense of internal disintegration. In Andrew, *all* his mental reality, all subjectivity had to be actively supported and protected from the invasion of anything that would be incompatible with it. He had to separate himself from *reality* and affirm his mentality, which caused constant tension. Although he fell into a vicious circle, he did not want to give up this situation, because only this gave him a sense of identity and self-worth. He did not note that he built his subjective paradise at the expense of living an illusion, at the expense of ignoring the real nature of the world and people. When he decided to go to psychotherapy, his activity in the world was limited to basic functions, he lived on a pension, and he experienced each requirement of the outside world as a deadly attack on himself.

This *real* led him to fury; when he was in contact with it, he did not find any point of support. Every human is torn between what is rational and what is irrational, between the understandable and predictable, and the unforeseen and inconceivable. Most people handle it somehow. However, Andrew— governed by the history of his life and perhaps other factors—chose only one pole, the pole of predictability and logicality. To put it in other words: he chose the idea, the pattern, and gave up life. This choice manifested itself in many ways. Andrew said he was "to some extent a heroic man," meaning his "consistency" and his "principles." His "heroism" (which to a certain degree was real heroism) manifested itself in his fight against *reality* and persistent following his own model of life. He said that he was "inept," but "capable of great emotions," that his "existence cannot keep up with his emotions." He often referred to his brother and other people as self-interested, able to do whatever it takes to achieve their goals. And he described himself as a sincere, emotional and honest person. He claimed to be "great in spirit" to listen to "great music," and he was worried that although he had been "raised on *The Trilogy*,[23] *Robinson Crusoe*, great music," he behaved the way he behaved, that is, he swore and had uncontrolled tics.

The inability to consciously feel guilt was characteristic of Andrew. Although he could admit that he had done wrong, breaking contact with his children, although he admitted his mistakes and said that he "took all the blame on himself," in the core of his identity, he remained perfect. This is best illustrated by the following situation. Andrew escorted a drunk friend home, and when he left him alone for a moment, the friend disappeared. It turned out that the man entered the road and got killed in a car accident. Andrew emphasized that he was "totally responsible for this death" and that he would "have to live with this until the end of his life." He said: "Someone else would bury their head in the sand, and I don't—I'm guilty and I won't hide it, I'm proud that I can take the blame on myself." Of course, he did not feel truly guilty. To feel guilty means to feel somewhat inferior, weakened, inadequate. Andrew did not feel that way—he felt most of all proud.

Similarly, he did not feel truly guilty against his children. He excluded these feelings from the sphere of his *ego*, which invariably remained "proud," "lofty," "subtle." He seemed to be detached from whatever bad he said about himself. Generally speaking, he eliminated the meaning of any life reality, which is not just our reference to it, but it means something in itself (e.g., if I kill someone, the most important thing is the fact that this person is dead, not that I understand my mistake). Reality did not function in the consciousness of his *ego*, but it emerged from the unconscious in the form of the punishing, self-destructive impulses.

This case shows one more thing. Identifying the obsessive remorse (of the *superego*) with morality, and the neurotic sense of guilt with guilt as understood by ethics, makes no sense. Catholic publicists sometimes state that psychotherapy unduly rids patients of guilt, putting the individual's well-being above ethics. Unfortunately, their considerations arise on the ground of complete ignorance of clinical issues. The areas of neurotic and ethical guilt are probably not disjunctive; their interrelationship is extremely complicated. Psychotherapy does not consist in—as these authors would like to see it— "absolving" the person whose "conscience is awakened" and making him indifferent to the ethical dimension. Nothing of the kind. Neuroticism is always an escape from the real confrontation with one's own guilt and responsibility.

Andrew's compulsions focused on the body, especially on the genitalia, eyes and hair, and he was constantly worried about them. He "checked" or "made sure" he had not hit his eye, damaged the genitalia with a knife, or polluted his hair with a harmful substance every single moment. "Checking" consisted in repeating the activity, which was the source of the alleged threat (e.g., he waved a knife around the crotch to "check" if the previous accidental movement could have injured it, he repeated the same movement for the same purpose around the eye about—as he counted himself—three thousand times).

The fact that Andrew's compulsions focused on these parts of the body was not a coincidence. Andrew had trouble with his eyesight, he was losing his hair, and was sensitive about his sexual prowess. All these spheres reminded him of the passage of time and aging. Andrew could not afford aging because he was constantly in the "before real life" phase; he was waiting for real love and passion. He never fully reached the stage of genital maturity, he was still a child that was about to enter the real world. He had specific feelings about dirty and dangerous objects and substances harmful to health. When he passed a dump, saw a toilet brush, or dog droppings, he felt that he was "attacked" as if these things were touching his head. He had the impression that he was attracted by these objects, and in the toilet he felt almost pressure on his head, pushed towards the toilet bowl, brush, or washing powder. He was afraid of knives that could harm his genitals.

These sensations intensified especially when he felt well and found himself attractive (for example after visiting the hairdresser). At some point during the psychotherapy (conducted in a sitting position), he started to have the impression that he touched the floor with his head. It shows that he, in a strange way, lost the sense of distance between himself and the outside world. Separated from reality, living in his own mind, he was now exposed to completely absurd attacks, as if reality had become particularly malicious. This can be understood as a sign of the unconscious counterbalance to his attitude of distancing himself.

He did not keep toothpastes, soaps, or any toiletries in the bathroom so that they were not near the toilet bowl. If, for example, he had stained his shoe with dog stool, the item became "contaminated" forever, no matter how thoroughly it was cleaned. He stored such "contaminated" things in one room, away from the bedroom. When the gas lighter fell on the floor, he grabbed it through a nylon bag. In this way, he "split" his surroundings into a clean and safe sphere and a dirty and threatening one. The more he isolated himself and the more he desired perfection and peace, the more he had to reject everything that was chaotic, accidental, and emotionally difficult. However, it did not help him to dispose of the unwanted impulses; quite the contrary—it intensified them.

Obviously, it was not the knife that could be dangerous, but his impulses. They were so uncontrollable that they could push his hand to grasp the knife and stab it into the body. His psyche transformed this situation into something opposite—into the sense of a threat from knives or harmful substances. It was them trying to attack him, not him wanting to attack himself with the use of these items. Naturally, it made him feel more secure, because he could avoid these objects. Andrew wanted to live in his own predictable and peaceful world, immersed in fantasy and contemplation of music. However, the outside world, along with his uncontrollable inner one, constantly invaded this paradise. Andrew could not stand it, wishing for absolute freedom and self-appeasement. When he felt that he could not keep his "over-happy" *self*, that he would be enslaved by the remaining sphere of his personality and the outside world, an impulse for self-destruction was born in him. He would be able to destroy himself rather than accept the imperfection of his human existence and the chaotic nature of the world. Although he was very sensitive about his health, and it was difficult for him to encounter any health problem, he fantasized of a deadly illness that would eventually free him from the torment of self-care, constant tension, and failures in the pursuit of absolute independence.

As a child, Andrew felt pushed away by his mother, and her role was largely taken over by his aunt. She was the only woman with whom he felt really connected all his life. Until the age of nine, during holidays, he slept with the aunt in one bed. Staying with the strange woman, who at the same time became the closest, must have triggered sexual feelings in him, but Andrew strongly denied that possibility. He defended himself against these feelings through the extreme idealization of his aunt and producing very sublime feelings for her. He took an almost idolatrous attitude towards her. Andrew idealized her and the relationship with her. Similarly, he idealized other women, but when he started a close relationship with any of them, he had to destroy this perfect image. He could not be tender to his female partners and desire them at the same time, because it would destroy his fantasies of tenderness and intimacy through what is *real* (lust, sex). This would threaten his imaginary relationship with his aunt, so important to his psychological balance. He did not combine love and desire also because it could make the repressed sexual feelings toward his aunt return, which would ruin the image too.

After his aunt's death he stopped oral sex, not to "sully" his lips with which he kissed her in the coffin. At that time, while making love to a woman, he had the aunt's face before his eyes, which made him sexually blocked. He unconsciously identified the partner with his aunt, whom he secretly desired as a child (imagining that St. Mary was naked was a similar return of the repressed impulse).

He said, with tenderness, that his shoes were "wonderful," because he wore them when visiting his aunt's grave and they "stood on the ground that covered her." "When they wear out, I'll take care of them, I won't throw them away"—he said as if he had described someone close. He was very attached to various objects, and behaved at home like a museum curator. This specific fetishism is the other side of intolerance of the *real*. In this way, Andrew symbolically "owned" these material artifacts, attributing special meaning to them. Things could not exist in an ordinary manner, they became either relics, in which the element of positive meaning prevailed, or contaminated things, carriers of equally defined but negative meanings (he also worshipped words, memories, dates).

Andrew made periodic attempts to isolate from his parents but was still emotionally dependent on them. During one session after my vacation, he spoke about his idea to stop the therapy, the decision to isolate from his "unreliable" parents, and the rebellion against God.[24] He treated the figure of God in a very concrete way. He wanted His tangible protection, but lost faith when feeling frustrated. God was to shelter him from the world, from its reality. If He did not do it, Andrew tried to achieve it himself. This happened after his friend lost his life, when he wanted to see the accident, for which he was in fact not responsible (at most co-responsible), as entirely his fault. In this way he turned his weakness and the accidentality of events into a sense of potency and meaning. Objecting to the existence of an accident, he often memorized the dates of unlucky events, tried to find causal relationships between coincidences, etc.

## Captivated by God—Clinical Case Study

Christopher's obsessions began in his childhood, when his parents sent him to a sanatorium for several months. He felt that things were going badly between his parents, and indeed, they soon separated. They probably sent the child to the sanatorium to spare him the distress, or maybe to avoid additional trouble. Whatever it was, it was a very hard time for Christopher. During therapeutic sessions, when he did not address the present issues, he constantly reverted to that period. He said then, bitterly resentful, that "the sanatorium sucked." The first obsessive thought he remembered was: "W. (his hometown) is there, Daddy is there, Mommy is there," he repeated it before he fell asleep. As he repeated the words, he was looking out the window in the direction in which his city was supposed to be. After he returned from the sanatorium, when the parents told him about their divorce, he began to stutter overnight. He was then sent to a children's camp for a few weeks. His obsessions grew over many years, until probably all of his daily activities became ritualized.

We can identify three groups of pathological behaviors in this case: rituals, compulsive attachment to order, and obsessive blasphemous thoughts together with the ones that were to negate them. Christopher's rituals focused mainly on the number two, some on the number five. One of them concerned the number seven and consisted in pressing the watch button seven times right after he woke up. Christopher tried to do everything twice: when he turned off the light, he switched it on and off again; he washed his socks, hung them on the radiator, then washed them again. The washing itself involved washing one of the socks five times, then the other, and then he repeated the whole sequence from the beginning. When he hit one foot, he did the same with the other, symmetrically. When one of his crutches fell (he walked with the help of crutches after a suicide attempt—he had jumped from a height), he dropped the other one. Leaving the house, he closed the door, opened it, and closed it again. If he made a hole in a sleeve, he stitched it together, but additionally trimmed the correspondent place on the second sleeve. When he closed the refrigerator or the wardrobe, he touched the door again (it was probably a substitute for double closing). He also felt the compulsion to double-tap his forehead. He tried to mask many of his activities, being aware that other people find them absurd. He tried to "avoid" the number three, because—as he claimed—this was the "number of Satan" (he referred to the symbol "666"). If he was to turn off the TV or radio, he waited for a "good" word and never turned off hearing a "bad" one (the examples of the "good" words included: "father," "pleasant aroma"; the "bad" ones were: "devil," "Satan," "murder"). Similarly, when he shelved the newspaper, or even turned the page, he had to look at a word or an illustration with positive connotations.

Christopher felt that if he stopped his rituals, something "terrible" would happen—with him, with me, or maybe "the whole world would collapse." When he heard in the media that a plane had crushed, he had the impression that he had contributed to it. Maybe he neglected some of his activities? All his things had to be carefully arranged and he always knew where he had put any of them. He particularly cared for symmetry: the alarm clock had to be placed exactly in the middle of the table, he put the crutches in line with the wall, and when he closed the drawer in the refrigerator, he did it with two fingers, so that each end was equally closed.

Another group of behaviors included those associated with religious symbols. Already in childhood, Christopher had to compulsively look at every religious picture or cross hung in the room, thinking the words, "God is here." In adult life, he still had to "tick off" each of the pictures this way. When he looked at the picture, he always uttered some formula, such as "Beloved God." At the same time, he was aware of the existence of the other stream of thoughts, in which he cursed God, using the worst words. He used various epithets for the crucified Jesus, such as "horse head" or "knight" (if the figure was cast in metal).

When Christopher saw the cross, he had to fold his hands as if in prayer, having an aversion to this symbol at the same time ("because I have to constantly pray to Him, fold these hands"). The blasphemy against God and the saints was what tormented Christopher the most, leading him to despair. He tried to overcome the curses that penetrated his consciousness by saying words of praise in his mind. He often spent many hours praying and expecting to be able to end the prayer to God with an affirmation. However, the most terrible blasphemies pushed into his mind. He began to pray more and more loudly, finally he started to cry and shout out words like "F. . . it all!"

Christopher lived in between the total dependence on the image of God and its extreme negation. When he prayed, he could never—and did not even want to—concentrate on prayer. Even when he did not blaspheme, he was distracted anyway, and was constantly thinking about something else. Whether he folded his pants well, whether he washed something or not. However, he could not give up his daily prayers, as if there was a correlation: the more superficial and mechanical the prayer was, the more necessary it was.

In interpersonal relations, Christopher functioned in a similar way. On the one hand, he was overly polite, and on the other, he often insulted his companion in his mind. During psychotherapeutic sessions, for example, he happened to call me "pal," for which he immediately apologized. However, this was not accidental. In this way he expressed the negation of the figure that he affirmed for other reasons. This behavior resulted from the fact that the fear Christopher experienced attached him in an extreme way to the figures he perceived as affecting his life. On the other hand, thanks to his blasphemous thoughts, he compensatively gained freedom. Originally, the figures he loved, on whom he was dependent, and who failed him were his parents.

Christopher's problem—just like the previous case—shows the essence of obsessive-compulsive disorder as an attempt to stop the flow of things and establish a phantasmatic, unchangeable reality. Christopher's activities gave him a seemingly unchanging existence. Christopher made everything stay at its own, always the same place, kept everything around him in order and symmetry (arrangement of the objects, the same wear of both crutches, etc.). What is symmetrical does not have a "resultant" that could be an impulse for movement and change, which is why it is static (see Weyl 1997, 19–21). Christopher achieved symmetry also in another way. Trying to pair each action—to add a mirror image, so to say—he received a kind of symmetry. A paired activity creates a symmetrical structure, a dyad which is associated with greater stability than oneness.[25]

Christopher's actions were specific—to use the term of geometry as a metaphor—automorphic transformations, that form an identical figure. In this way, although he was active in the world, he avoided changes and evolution. Compulsive counting was also supposed to maintain some semblance of control over reality. No action could be accidental, so he could not afford actions he did not count (for example, he could not rinse the glass a random number of times). Why was any lack of such "control" over reality threatening? Because it involved a vision of destruction of the *ego* by revealing what is *beyond-the-ego*, and thus is *real*. The obsessive "rationality" was to protect against self-destruction, which was a compensatory response of the repressed part of his personality to the falseness of his *ego*. As in the previous case, Christopher denied all guilt and mistake, wishing to keep the happy *ego*. The reality of his life—real desires and sense of guilt—was pushed beneath the threshold of his consciousness, and from there attacked his false identity.

Christopher was afraid that if he stopped performing his rituals, "the world would collapse." The ritual was to keep the existence of the world and its order. When he addressed God, he always asked Him to "make everything OK," and he did not dare think about any particular request. Why? Because thinking about a particular danger evoked anxiety. We deal here with the immanent aspect of obsessive-compulsive disorder, which is the attempt to maintain certain fantasies and a certain point of view, that would be threatened by a fuller view of reality. It is not just about the usual fear of danger, the "fear of death." It is about the fear of the *ego*, as a self-aware mental structure, of *reality*.

Christopher's *ego* was so fragile that it was afraid to take *reality* into consideration. He felt that his prayers were a kind of "forcing" God to answer them. For this reason, he called himself an "egoist" (some elements of his relation to God are similar to those in the previous case—these elements are characteristic of obsessive-compulsive disorder in general). Indeed, although he meant well for the whole world (he wished there would be no wars, no air crashes), he really meant his own safety that could be guaranteed only by a calm and unchanging world.

Christopher had a specific sense of magical influence on reality. He believed that natural disasters, accidents, also happy events were associated with his activities. He did not describe this influence in a psychotic way, he did not insist on its existence. However, the affective level turned out to be stronger and Christopher functioned as if he had been completely certain that these dependencies existed. What was the function of these beliefs? Although he lived in anxiety and tension provoked by the idea that so much depended on his actions, in this way he placed himself in the center of the world events and gained control over reality. By taking this pathological position, he could keep the fantasy of the orderly and nonautonomous world that was, so to speak, "focused" on him (in childhood he felt totally powerless and probably wanted power; now he thought he had it).

Turning away from reality and domination of mental representations make reality divide into the chaotic *materia prima* and the opposing *nomos* of the mind. In his experience, the patient oscillates between these poles. If he can secure his mental peace by means of a ritual, the world becomes an overly ordered cosmos. If the protective function of the ritual fails, the *ego* gets attacked by the irrational chaos.

## NOTES

1. "Neurosis," "neuroticism" are the concepts that are not included in the latest version of the *DSM-5* (*Diagnostic and Statistical Manual of Mental Disorders*); currently one refers to "disorders" (anxiety disorder, obsessive-compulsive disorder, etc.). But the notion of neurosis—besides the fact that it has a long tradition and is

still used by psychiatrists—is heuristically useful, being a collective term for a certain group of problems.

2. As we saw above, Freud also equated neurosis with individual religiosity.

3. I prescind from the fact that the term "schizophrenia" created by Eugen Bleuler did not appear until 1908. Cases of psychosis had been described, of course, much earlier.

4. I do not understand, however, why Hoevels says that if Freud showed that religion is a collective neurosis, it is now necessary to examine what form of individual neurosis it corresponds with (Hoevels 1997, 229), since Freud clearly said that it is the obsessional neurosis (Freud 1961b, 43).

5. In psychiatry, psychotherapy or psychoanalysis, "neuroses," "personality disorders," "character types" are mentioned. The distinction between neurotic disorders and personality disorders is often half-intuitive. It can be said that, in general, personality disorders are characterized by greater ego-syntonicity (consistency with the *ego*) than neuroses, which means that the individual does not directly feel the discomfort caused by the symptoms. His behavior is integrated with the whole personality, and often the environment suffers more than the patient himself. In this case, rather, the whole character is a "symptom" that the person has learned to live with and may not even notice it. In the case of neurosis, there is greater dynamism, the *ego* is plagued by symptoms that are something alien to the patient, something that tortures him and that he would like to get rid of. Also, in the case of personality disorders, one may be aware of the problem, but often it is only shown by the reaction of the environment. In neurosis, one feels more clearly that "there is something wrong with him." The character type is still normal, although it shows some similarity to the corresponding personality disorder.

6. Weber, unlike Marx, argues that the ideas shaped before can have a decisive influence on the development of relations of production. He shows that the mentality of the Puritans and the Pietists, formed in an atmosphere of rationality and respect for work, underlie the explosion of the capitalist economy.

7. There are also inconsistencies. Perhaps Protestantism is not less "communal" than Catholicism—from a certain angle it may be considered to be more community-focused. The pastor's words always refer to the congregation (the community of worshippers), whereas in the Catholic mass the congregation of the faithful was originally not of primary importance, for a mass was first of all a symbolic presentation of the sacrifice of Christ (until the Second Vatican Council in the 1960s). Similarly, the Protestant common songs, lectures, and sermons are supposed to have a significant impact on the social life of the community, as opposed to more "symbolic" Catholic sermons. It is an open question to what extent the language of female mystics is coincident with hysteria through the sexualization of experiences, and to what extent it is something opposite through the full expression of erotic feelings, since in hysteria they are in principle not fully experienced. It is also worth considering to what degree Catholic dogmatics, through deliberately keeping areas of mystery and tolerating contradictions, ascends the heights of thought, and how close it is to hysterical reasoning.

8. This is Freud's first version of the dualistic theory of drives. Later, Freud revised the theory, introducing the conflict between the life and death drives in place of

the original distinction. He considered the second theory to be the final one. I believe that the second metapsychological theory of drives does not absorb or replace the first one. In my opinion, both these theories contain the elements that should be regarded as complementary (meaning: only the third theory could combine and replace them).

9. In biology, there is a dispute over the subject of this "second law," i.e., whether the reproductive instinct serves the species, lineage, or gene (see Dawkins 2016a).

10. Evolutionary psychology also concentrates on the non-individual side of man; it assumes that human behavior results not so much from individualized motivations, but from unconscious programs that have evolved in the course of evolution. These programs are not to serve the individual, but the "reproductive success" (see Buss 2016). An extreme expression of the approach that diminishes the importance of a single organism—i.e., that emphasizes the second biological law—is seeing the individual as a simple "gene vehicle" (Dawkins 2016b).

11. Throughout the book, I use my own model of the human psyche, which I perceive as involved in the conflict between the totalizing and separating nature of consciousness and the necessity to exist in broader natural and interpersonal systems. Man is neither the consciousness contemplating itself, free from the outside world, nor the world's fully assimilated part without identity. He constantly oscillates between these poles, unable to choose any of them. Thus, in the structure of the human psyche there is a conflict between being an individual and being a moment in the time and space extent of the species. The human psyche is as much individualized as collective. I use the term *coiling up* to define the force that strives for individualization, its product is, for instance, the *ego*. I define the collective element in the psyche as the area of *participation*. This area is not so largely subjected to volitional control as the *coiled up* part, and its domain is interpersonal relations.

12. The Oedipus complex, in the Freudian sense, consists in the child's sexual attachment to the parent of the opposite sex and more or less conscious aggression (expressed in the form of a death wish) towards the parent of the same sex. The child's struggle with emotions towards the dyad of parents is a fundamental process shaping the structure of personality (Rusbridger 2000, 1–9).

13. Perhaps the idea of love in general (as it is presented, for example, by Paul of Tarsus in *The First Letter to the Corinthians*) is in large part a phantasm created as a result of the reversal of human needs into [phantasmatic] fulfillment. Simply put: we want a lot more than we can get and give, but we have created a vision that all these needs will be satisfied.

14. The Bible presents not only the idea of the *ex nihilo* creation, but also forming or making (*yäcar*) man from the "dust of the earth" (*'afär*)—this seems to temper human narcissism.

15. Marx, the author of an elaborate theory of political economy, a great diagnostician of economic forces shaping culture, was known for being completely unable to balance his budget. He was in constant poverty and throughout all his creative life, he was financially supported by a friend of his, Friedrich Engels, who was closer to the realities of "practical economics." Of course, such facts do not negate the values of the work of both these authors, but they are a contribution to analyze it from the right perspective.

16. Since there are so many similarities between psychoanalytic therapy and the proletarian revolution, one can ask, why psychoanalysis would be (on the individual plane) more effective than revolution (in the social area), which, after all, proved to be a completely unsuccessful endeavor. I will risk an answer. The superiority of psychoanalysis results from: following the patient, the ability to constantly change one's judgments about him, and patience. The analyst can quickly get a general picture of the patient's problem and see a way of solving it. And yet, therapy always requires a long time. This is because working through the problem requires constant interaction with the patient, sensitivity to his words, and constant modification of interpretations. The Communist Party acted differently. It was to be the vanguard of the working class, its consciousness (Kołakowski 1976, vol. 2, 51–54, 457 et seq.). By definition, like the psychoanalyst, it was only meant to indicate, make aware of what takes place anyway (that is, the inevitable historical process of social change). However, it did otherwise—it lost contact with reality and instead of showing the social truth, it began to manipulate it, falsify it, and create its own. Candidates for psychoanalysts are trained and verified for a long time to avoid this.

17. Nietzsche's problems were ascribed to syphilis, neurosis, bipolar disorder. It was attempted to separate the period in which he was healthy from the time of collapse, madness. I see Nietzsche as a psychotic who after a period of relatively good social functioning broke down and fell into a state of manifest, clinical psychosis.

18. The Latin term *obsessio* is used by Christian demonology to describe the states of being harassed and disturbed by the evil spirit. The term "obsession" derives from it, indicating an obsessive thought. The term *possessio* means greater interference of the devil through overpowering, possession.

19. The latency stage (latency of sexual needs) is a term introduced by Freud to indicate the developmental phase in which sexual desires are inactive. This stage lasts from the end of early childhood to the time of puberty, i.e., from about 7 to 11–13 years of age (Moore and Fine 1996, 370–71).

20. This can be compared to the Lacanian understanding of the term "the Real." However, I use this concept in a slightly different sense. The insights presented in this book arose without knowing Jacques Lacan's theory, based on epistemological and psychopathological reflections, such as the issue of relativity of theories, the problem of language limitations (which refers to the issues that I discussed in chapter 1), and the accounts of patients with psychosis and obsessive-compulsive disorder. Originally, I spoke of "reality in itself," after getting acquainted with Lacan's terminology, I chose the term "the *real*" (and also "*reality*").

21. So we deal with manifestations of something that needs to be called an "unconscious sense of guilt." This concept is very important for the understanding of psychopathology in general, because it seems to play a role in the internal dynamics of almost all mental disorders. We say that the sense of guilt is "unconscious" because it does not manifest itself as a direct reflection, but is indirectly identified through the analysis of behaviors, statements, and events in the patient's life. We call it all a "sense" mainly for linguistic reasons, because by using the shorter phrase "unconscious guilt," we would suggest the existence of some objective state, whereas here it is the subjective one (Freud 1974, 123).

22. All the patients' names and identifying details have been changed in the book.

23. *The Trilogy*—a series of novels written by Henryk Sienkiewicz, a Polish author and Nobel Prize laureate.

24. This situation refers to the issue of the relationship between the figures of parents and the image and attitude toward God that I address in chapter 3.

25. In numerological systems, oneness is "male" and active, and dyad is "female" and passive.

*Chapter Three*

# Child, Parent, God

## EARTHLY PARENTS AND HEAVENLY GUARDIANS

### God in the Image of Father or Father in the Image of God?

Investigating the connections between neurosis and religion, one must not omit the issue of the relation between the image of parents and the formation of the cultural and individual vision of God. According to the model of neurosis presented above, a problematic relationship with parents and its psychological representation are the etiological elements of this disorder. In addition, in both cases of obsessive-compulsive disorder described above (they were selected randomly) the connection between experiencing the relationship with parents and the relation to God becomes overt. For Freud, the father played the main role in these processes:

> Religion would thus be the universal obsessional neurosis of humanity; like the obsessional neurosis of children, it arose out of the Oedipus complex, out of the relation to the father. (Freud 1961b, 43)

> The psychoanalysis of individual human beings, however, teaches us with quite special insistence that the god of each of them is formed in the likeness of his father, that his personal relation to God depends on his relation to his father in the flesh and oscillates and changes along with that relation, and that at bottom God is nothing other than an exalted father. As in the case of totemism, psychoanalysis recommends us to have faith in the believers who call God their father, just as the totem was called the tribal ancestor. If psychoanalysis deserves any attention, then—without prejudice to any other sources or meanings of the concept of God, upon which psychoanalysis can throw no light—the paternal element in that concept must be a most important one. (Freud 2004, 171)

Next, in the article entitled "A Seventeenth-Century Demonological Neurosis," in which he analyzes the case of Christoph Haizmann, a painter, Freud says:

> To begin with, we know that God is a father-substitute; or, more correctly, that he is an exalted father; or, yet again, that he is a copy of a father as he is seen and experienced in childhood—by individuals in their own childhood and by mankind in its prehistory as the father of the primitive and primal horde. Later on in life the individual sees his father as something different and lesser. But the ideational image belonging to his childhood is preserved and becomes merged with the inherited memory-traces of the primal father to form the individual's idea of God. (Freud 1961a, 85)

God is "nothing but an exalted father." Most likely, the majority of the faithful, when faced with this statement, want to immediately contradict. But although the above words cannot be accepted without reservations, one cannot just reject them. For psychological observation points to a number of facts that are close to Freud's radical conclusion. The influence of the parent-child relationship on the phenomenon of religiousness cannot be denied. What is hard to agree with is not psychological facts and Freud's observations, but their epistemological horizon. Freud, a genius whose conclusions are of great insight, in this case significantly narrowed down this horizon. This is, in my opinion, a rather strange situation, considering that he always weighed his words and underlined the temporariness and incompleteness of his knowledge of many issues. On the other hand, for example, Freud's following statement seems to indicate that his position was not so unambiguous:

> Thus we recognize that the roots of the need for religion are in the parental complex; the almighty and just God, and kindly Nature, appear to us as grand sublimations of father and mother, or rather as revivals and restorations of the young child's ideas of them. Biologically speaking, religiousness is to be traced to the small human child's long-drawn-out helplessness and need of help; and when at a later date he perceives how truly forlorn and weak he is when confronted with the great forces of life, he feels his condition as he did in childhood, and attempts to deny his own despondency by a regressive revival of the forces which protected his infancy. The protection against neurotic illness, which religion vouchsafes to those who believe in it, is easily explained: it removes their parental complex, on which the sense of guilt in individuals as well as in the whole human race depends, and disposes of it, while the unbeliever has to grapple with the problem on his own. (Freud 1957a, 123) [1]

So Freud sees the positive function of religion. It is to enable the faithful to dispose of the parental complex, while the unbeliever has to cope with it in another way. But does the latter achieve something more? Does he, through his labors, achieve something that the believer does not have? Freud does not give an answer. His ultimate standpoint seems to be expressed in the following reasoning: since the image of God is associated with the situation of the child's helplessness and with the figure of the father as the one who gives shelter, it means it is produced from these elements. So "God" is nothing more than a product of infantilism, meaning He cannot exist for the truly mature consciousness.

Freud's radical rejection of theistic religion seems to contradict his ability to notice metascientific limitations of the constructed theories. It seems that the intensity of this aversion to religion would itself demand a psychoanalytic interpretation (Freud had an exceptionally ambivalent attitude to religion—he intensively and thoroughly dealt with it and, at the same time, ruthlessly negated its value; see Meissner 1984, 21 et seq.). I think that there is some vagueness in Freud's view of religion. Does religion ultimately eliminate the parental complex or does it become its preservative? Or maybe it transforms it in a specific way? Freud saw various functions of religion, which could not be directly reduced to infantilism and illusion, but in his considerations he did not sufficiently allow for this aspect.

By reducing the importance of religion, Freud did not take into account that it concerns existentially inevitable elements; being mortal, it is impossible not to be longing (for care). So his negation of the solutions suggested by religion, even if they are just phantasmatic, is not a significant achievement. Man, made aware this way, does not become stronger. Taking into account our existential situation, the nature of our being as being-through-caretakers, we can reach a completely different conclusion. I would say that God and parents are so close to each other in the human psyche that they *seem* to be one. Rudolf Otto put it this way:

> So, too, the phrase "We ought to fear, love, and trust him" is verbally identical, whether it refers to the relation of child to father or to that of man to God. But again in the second case these ideas are infused with a meaning of which none but the religious-minded man can have any comprehension or indeed any inkling, whose presence makes, e.g., the "fear of God" "something more" than any fear of a man, qualitatively, not merely quantitatively, though retaining the essence of the most genuine reverence felt by the child for its father. (Otto 1958, 47)

This complicated aspect was also expressed by Jung, when he said that transformation of the libido into the archetypal image is:

> a universal phenomenon which forms the basis of all our ideas of God, and these are so old that one cannot tell whether they are derived from a father-imago, or vice versa. (The same must be said of the mother-imago as well.) (Jung 1976, 60)

So it is about a fundamental moment, very difficult to analyze rationally. I believe the contradiction must be maintained to get closer to the truth. We need to keep in mind all the empirical findings of psychology regarding the relation between the figures of parents and the image and idea of God, as well as the specificity and "absoluteness" of this idea.

To illustrate this approach, we can refer to the research of Stanislav Grof, one of the authors of transpersonal psychology (Grof 1985). It does not directly concern the "parent-God" issue, but religious ideas in general. Grof proved that visionary experiences after taking LSD are arranged in thematic groups that correspond to the great images of religion, such as paradise, hell, judgment, or resurrection. At the same time, they correlate with four perinatal phases (fetus in the uterus—first contractions—birthing with passing through the birth canal—birth). One can therefore conclude that all these visions result from perinatal experiences, and religion and mysticism are poetic images of childbirth.

And yet Grof points out that the psychological and transpersonal processes we discover here go beyond the reality of childbirth (Grof 1988). Experiences during a psychedelic session or holotropic breathing are not reduced to the biology of birth. But do we know what a birth is? How does the birth of a single man connect with the births of other people, the births of mammals, and the "births" of all life on Earth? We enter the mystery of our existence here. Do we know the beginning of life? The root of the universe?

Nothing precludes the issue of reproduction and birth from reaching the "absolute." And it can be similar with the categories of parenthood, motherhood, and fatherhood that underlie the image of the deities.

### Religion—for or against Neurosis?

The general approach to neuroticism implies the conclusion that the neurotic personality has a special propensity to seek consolation outside, in stronger powers. Every neurotic is a potential worshipper and follower, because he makes his well-being dependent on external support more than others. The support he expects regards in principle a "solution" to his earthly fate, so a kind of "salvation." However, clinical observation does not indicate that neurotics particularly actively belong to religious groups, especially often pray or sit in the first pew in church. Perhaps their "religions" are more internal, unstable, pagan? Religiousness as such does not need to be a preservative of an immature attitude to life, but it may equally well be a factor that makes it possible to achieve self-reliance and accept greater responsibility for one's own life. Widely understood, faith (in God and eternal life, reincarnation, higher purpose, metaphysical justice, or another kind of legitimization of one's own existence) seems to be sometimes the only factor that can save the individual from chronic psychological pathology.

Recall what we said about neurosis. We described the neurotic as a mentally dependent person. The neurotic lives as if he divided people into two separate groups: *parents* and *children*. He himself is a child, so he expects to find a *parent* who will help him. The *parent* is to be his earthly savior. If he does not find him, he falls into despair. And yet the Christian religion leaves no illusions here, saying that man should not place his hopes in people. By showing the misery of man, it makes people equal. Thus, it stops the neurotic looking around. Man already knows that he will not find what he needs among people. But the need does not disappear, it only goes beyond the social world, into the "heavenly" realm. This vertical shift can be an extension of consciousness, a kind of break out of the ties of the child's past. How is such a view of religion different from Freud's claims? Freud argued that the persistence of the sense of dependence, fear of the world, and looking for comfort beyond oneself is a manifestation of the still lasting infantile feelings one should have rid himself of long ago. In my opinion, it is impossible to divest oneself of these feelings. However, they can be transformed, projected beyond the social world just to make it possible for the individual to take a realistic attitude towards it. For Freud, the image of God preserved infantile feelings towards one's own parents. As a father-substitute, it was the cause of maintaining the immature attitude in adulthood. But what if the image of God can, for some people, become the only salvation from the image of parents that is overwhelming and infantilizing, and its influence is impossible to annihilate?

## Dependence on Parents and the Archetype of Divinity

Each of us has parents and each of us was once a child. This statement is a truism, but keeping it in mind may make it possible to better understand many issues related to human life, including religious life. The Jews, when they heard of Jesus's teaching, said, "And they said, Is not this Jesus, the son of Joseph, whose father and mother we know? how doth he now say, I am come down out of heaven?" (John 6:42). In the Gospel of Mark, as a continuation of the parallel theme, Jesus answers, "And Jesus said unto them, A prophet is not without honor, save in his own country, and among his own kin, and in his own house. And he could there do no mighty work, save that he laid his hands upon a few sick folk, and healed them" (Mark 6:4–5). According to Judaism, "when the Christ cometh, no one knoweth whence he is" (John 7:27).

The above-mentioned words reveal an important psychological mechanism that links "divinity" and the issue of the parent-child relationship. For God cannot have parents. The true God's parent can only be God alone, with whom the Son is "coessential." Catholic theology, which that strives for a higher cognition through maintaining contradictions, keeps the relation of sonship and fatherhood and at the same time makes both "persons" equal. Thus, we equally have and do not have a parental relationship here. In any case, it is not a relationship that we could directly associate with one we know from nature. As we can see from the Bible quotes, having known parents weakens the child's power. Knowing the genesis of the individual, that is his family of origin, lessens his power. For the Savior comes from nowhere, He is a "self-made man" and an "eternal adult."

Let us recall the frequent images of the infant Jesus as a "mini-adult" whose face displays intelligence and self-awareness. Similarly, the Buddha is said to have been born fully conscious. It is no different in the case of the heroes of Greek mythology, such as Heracles or Hermes, or many other religious figures. As for the earthly parents of divine or deified persons, they are usually moved into the background. According to Christian theology, Joseph is in no sense Jesus's father. And the Buddha's mother was impregnated by a small elephant that entered her side (Chiodo 2002, 21–22). We observe a similar mechanism in most religions and even within the mythologization of history. The legendary founders of Rome, Romulus and Remus, were born of a mother impregnated by the god Mars (Eliade 1994a, 75). Next, according to Diogenes Laertius who refers to other ancient authors, there were rumors in Athens that "divine" Plato's father, Ariston, wanted to rape Perictione, the future philosopher's mother. However, he did not manage to do it, and when Apollo appeared in his dream, he did not get near her until the child was born (Diogenes 2018, 134). Olympias, Alexander the Great's mother, is said to have been impregnated by a god in the form of a serpent (Plutarch 2004, 4). Plutarch writes that:

> Once [. . .] a serpent was found lying by Olympias as she slept, which more than anything else, it is said, abated Philip's passion for her; whether he feared her as an enchantress, or thought she had commerce with some god, and so looked on himself as excluded, he was ever after less fond of her conversation. (Plutarch 2004, 4)

Apollo is also said to be the father of the emperor Octavian Augustus, who during his lifetime sought for his deification (Jaczynowska 1987, 116–17). Sargon, Moses, Cyrus escaped from the power of their parents (at least the real ones). Each of these examples shows a detachment of a given person from his family roots, from the psychologically indelible period of dependence on his omnipotent caregivers. When one succeeds, he automatically gains power. The fact that it usually concerns the father results from realities. It is equally necessary for the god to detach himself from the mother—the future Buddha deliberately chose a mother who was supposed to die seven days after his birth (Chiodo 2002, 21); Jesus renounced his relationship with his mother (Matthew 12:46–50, Mark 3:31–35, Luke 8:19–21). So if gods have mothers, it is also because the thought that someone may be created without her is usually too unrealistic.

The need to detach the deity from the parents is determined by the archetypal image of power that springs from self-existence and independence. However, each child, dependent on his or her parents and influenced by the Oedipus complex and the family structure, is deprived of this power. Although the personal development of a person is closely related to his independence from his parents, the fact is that this independence is never complete. According to Freud, the Oedipus complex is the core of every neurosis. What does it mean? Well, neurosis is an expression of our maladjustment to the conditions of the world. And what underlies it, what builds its shape, is the nature of our attitude towards parents. As I have already mentioned, we can consider the Oedipus complex as a detailed manifestation of the general parental complex, which is the intrapsychic sum of dependence on parents, the whole satisfaction and frustration resulting from the relationship with them. A therapist who has the opportunity to clearly see its strength, can also see a new image of the individual. It is a "nonautonomous" person whose psyche exists in relation to the figures of his parents. They are in the structure of the psyche more than just images of memory—they are parts of this structure. Parents are not only "remembered," but constitute a "substructure" of the child's psychic structure. In his experiencing, the patient constantly, consciously and unconsciously, refers to the figures of his caregivers. He does not only "think about them," but also "is the thinking about them." He is never fully independent, and his parents—more precisely: their mental representations—constantly affect his life.

So the psyche of every human being is inscribed in the infinite line of previous generations, never being a fully self-existent entity. This kind of "insolvability" of the parental complex is an existential fact of our life—concrete biographical and psychological determinants are only modifications of this basic and unavoidable component of the human condition.

The psychological dependence of man clearly expresses itself in the phenomenon of transference that develops in the course of psychotherapy. In the process of so-called transference neurosis,[2] the patient mentally sticks to the therapist, considering him as a mana figure.[3] His symptoms, mood, sense of meaning or meaninglessness of life—all these elements—become modifiable by the therapist, or more precisely by how the patient perceives the therapist at a given moment. If, for example, he finds him strong, attentive and close, he feels that there is hope for him, that he can face the world. In moments of doubt, when the therapeutic process brings in distance, he may feel that he is completely lonely and powerless. Psychotherapy leads the patient from support and dependence, through various frustrations, to self-reliance. However, this is a long-lasting process and it is difficult to say how many cases end with the full resolution of the transference, when the patient begins to see that the therapist is an equally defective human being, without simultaneously negating the effects of the therapy.

Generally, transference, along with its psychophysical effects, shows how superficial the subjective cohesion and autonomy are. Transference neurosis develops as the psyche seeks to repeat the childhood situation, with its pathological aspects. In adults, psychological structures formed within childhood relationships with parents are the factors that affect behavior the most. For a child, the parent is the real Absolute. He or she is the creator and master of the child's world. This is why the early childhood conditioning and the power of childhood traumas are of such great weight. The parent's voice is God's voice, and the parent's actions have a cosmic significance, because a small child does not have any place where he or she could hide from the parent's sight, decision, and influence. The child in relation to the parent is like Job in his relationship with God. When the parent is not good enough, the child cannot simply turn away, but must stay. The child cannot find itself any compensating relationship with another person. Even if it was possible physically, which in the case of a small child is an absurd assumption, it is completely out of the question psychologically. After all, the child does not even know what a relationship is. It is the parent who shows it to the child, who cannot even imagine the distance from the "bad" parent because he or she does not know anyone else or any other relationship. When we are adults, and someone annoys us, seems bad or stupid, we can oppose him, leave him, or negate him in our mind. Such actions are always based on the confidence that there are good, wise, and friendly people. Therefore, meeting such a person is usually not a tragedy for us. However, the child is in a completely different position—if he or she has a "bad" parent, there is no way out.

We said that independence from parents is never possible to a full extent. However, if it does not take place to a basic degree, the person will never be free and responsible for himself. Dependence on parents can occur on many levels: emotional, financial, related to all kinds of help on their part, or just the opposite—it can be associated with a conviction resulting from a symbiotic relationship that the parents constantly need the child. It can be overt or hidden. One can be dependent on the parents he lives with, as well as on their images that are carried in himself, although the real contact does not exist for a long time.

Becoming independent of parents is a long-term process, perhaps always unfinished. Psychotherapy invariably reveals "incomplete figures"—to use the expression of Gestalt therapy—in our relationships with parents. The representations of these unresolved conflict relations, located deep inside our psyche, constantly affect our current situation, manifesting themselves in the form of a more or less evident compulsion to repeat.[4] Individuals that may seem fully autonomous display the strength with which their parents continue to influence their lives only during psychotherapy. Their inner "child" (the affective-cognitive complex hidden in the unconscious, which is the heritage of childhood) is constantly subjected to them. No one considered to have divine power, to be a mythical or mythologized figure, can afford such a lack of autonomy. This is because it is this figure to be the start, to create the future, without the ballast of the past. In the case of a normal person, everything begins in the past, in a situation created by the parents, whose lives were influenced by their parents, who had their own parents, etc. During psychotherapy, the patient tries to reach this darkness of his own prehistory and control it. It seems, however, that it never becomes fully possible. Therefore, man must remain with what is not his.

## The Marcionist Phantasm

Each of us has come across older authority figures. Some of them are like moving statues, whose almost every gesture seems to have a symbolic dimension. We often feel like children when in contact with such people. In these cases, our *ego*—following the conceptualization of Eric Berne's transactional analysis—involuntarily enters the Child state (Berne 1973).[5] We feel physically and intellectually inferior, less important than usual. If we do not become adorers of the persona endowed with "power"—which can become a source of our own strength—we will definitely be doomed to a moment of mental discomfort. These people usually deliberately adopt and keep the image, because it is a gateway to their self-esteem and a way to deal with other people.

What can we do to change this unpleasant situation? For example, we can imagine that this sage, ruler, or hero was once an infant, just like us. He needed his mother's tender care, he cried of hunger, he could not satisfy any of his needs himself. His caregivers were everything to him, and their power over him was practically unlimited. They could let him survive without major wounds, or they could cause scars that he would never rid himself of. Although we now see this man as the incarnation of the father archetype, he is not the father of himself. He has a father and is his child. He is not the "absolute" father, as we would like to perceive him sometimes, but only a relative father, established within the fatherhood-sonship relationship. We, however—to a different degree—constantly seek an "absolute" parent. That is why we see ourselves so easily as someone worse, let others play their game and sometimes suffer because of this. We easily submit to the mechanism of projection of archetypal—and therefore ideal and not real—images onto certain people. It may seem to us then that we met a guru or master who fully controls his life. When this happens, our perception becomes stereotypical, we do not accept the information that does not match the idealized image. This is why Catholics react so emotionally to any modifications of the conventional image of the Holy Father. The same applies to the followers of other religions and cults when it comes to the images of their priests and gurus. Even the "followers" of some therapeutic approaches want to perceive their pioneers or prominent representatives in the same way. They are reluctant, however, to see any—except for the elements fitting the conventional image—genesis of the "great man." The followers would definitely not like to know that in his mind there are still some needs and weaknesses that formed when he did not think about "great things" yet.

A similar mechanism occurs in the functioning of children who often protest or cry when their parents become less "parental" in their eyes. This is the case, for example, when parents start fooling around. Just for their own amusement, not when playing with the child. The child seems to be threatened by the mere existence of the "non-parental" side of the parent. It behaves just as if it wanted the parent to be an *absolute parent*. This desire never disappears, because later, when we already know that our parents are not "absolute," we transfer it to other people. And further—to the image of God.

Having said this, the child's world is initially limited to the world that the parents create around it. The parents, due to their physical closeness, are the only people that the child clearly perceives, the people who constantly absorb its psyche. Over time, when the child matures, the circle of people and phenomena available to it expands, and it cognitively and behaviorally goes beyond the family. Now, the child can see the parents, who earlier seemed to be perfect and omnipotent, in a broader context. It becomes aware of the parents' imperfections and the fact that maybe the parents of other children are better, that is, they care more about their offspring, are more forgiving and devoted. The birth of younger siblings can be an additional factor here. This event and the changes resulting from it strengthen the child's sense of alienation even more.

In a situation where parents are no longer perceived as existing only for the child, and the desire for unconditional care lasts, a characteristic fantasy may arise, namely the idea that one is a foster child and the current caregivers are not real parents. These real parents are certainly better, more meaningful and respectable than the present caregivers who dared to call themselves "parents" (see Freud 1997a, 215–16).

This individual psychological dynamism shows significant convergence with one of the basic statements of Gnosticism, and in particular Marcionism, namely that God known to us is not the real God, but only an inferior demiurge, the creator of "this world." The true God is unknown to us, he is *deus otiosus*, whose existence is not easy to see. Marcion, who as a young man was excommunicated by his father bishop for unorthodox views (Rops 1997, 292), created the theology of "a better God" (Jonas 1994, 152–85). He claimed that this is a truly "good" God, not only "just," as Jewish Jehovah. This God is the father of Jesus Christ and calls us through him. It is characteristic of this type of speculation that this true, supreme God is completely "alien" to the world. Marcion, just like Gnostics, particularly emphasized this strangeness. It is an expression of majesty and power here. Gnostics denied the greatness of the world-God, and—like a child that rejects his or her real parents, imagining that there are better parents somewhere, that is, not entangled in the chaos of present relationships—believed in the existence of the God absolutely beyond the world. They claimed, however, that an inner spark connects us with this God, and that the human soul is close to God, being as alien to the world as He is. Marcion went further—he stated that both the whole world and the whole man are alien to God. Thus, he exalted the "father" even more, detaching him from absolutely everything that man can come into contact within or beyond himself. Looking at this matter from the perspective of the child's fantasies and needs—or from the perspective of infantile needs occurring in every adult—the father was exalted to the position of the longed-for *absolute father* whose life is completely different from the child's life. It is the father in no way related to what is infantile (meaning: earthly and human), thus offering a promise of maximum security. The relationship with someone like that can be extremely asymmetrical in the end—he is supposed to care, not needing any help himself. His life has no infantile (meaning: human) limitations. Only he, unlike a man-child, is truly omnipotent.

## FATHER, GOD, SATAN—CLINICAL CASE STUDY

I will now present the life story told by a patient—call her Joanna. I never met her in person. Her entire story was written down by the head nurse, completely independently of my investigations. This story was not triggered, the patient herself wished to share it. As we shall see, there is much about both the father and God in this story.

Joanna's story was subjected to an analysis as detailed as was possible in the case of an account written by someone else. Interpreting the suffering person's account is always morally sensitive, particularly when he or she talks about serious issues such as pain, defeat, or search for meaning in God. An interpretation may give the impression that we divest someone of his or her faith or deconstruct his or her God. Fortunately, we neither have such a right nor power, as human existence goes beyond any analysis.

Joanna was diagnosed with schizoaffective disorder.[6] When she came to the hospital, she was depressed, full of self-accusations and suicidal thoughts; she said she had lost her faith in God. Pharmacotherapy caused Joanna's behavior and mood to became manic, she became, in turn, psychomotorically agitated. She said then that she regained her faith in God and life. She began her story saying that she had loved her father as "senselessly" as a little girl. She said: "I felt safe in his arms, I knew that nothing would happen to me when he was there." She then went on to describe her family situation of the time she was a child.

Here is her entire account:

My father was seriously ill, I think he suffered from depression or he was crazy about cleaning. I saw him on his knees all the time, he was constantly cleaning something. He called us and our mother sons of a b . . . , he beat my brother unconscious. Then I pounded against the wall, I loved my brother very much. Father beat Mother in front of me. I remember the first time when I was three years old. He fed me on gruel and at the same time hit my mother on the head, with a plate. He smashed her head, she didn't defend herself. They left me alone at home; for example, they waited for me to fall asleep and left. I was scared to death. I howled at the door, our neighbors came and comforted me through the door. Then I went back to bed. I don't know how it happened, but when I was two or three years old, I discovered pleasure in touching myself. I started to masturbate as a few-year-old child and since then I've done it very often. I treated it as a medicine for loneliness, it gave me comfort and relaxation. Parents continued to fight. Mother was a complete loser, father humiliated her at every turn, even in people's presence. I hated her for it. He also called me names, beat my brother and locked him in the basement. Father started abusing me sexually when I turned ten. I had to wait for him in bed. He didn't rape me in the strict sense, but he touched me and I had to touch him. I disgusted him on the one hand, but on the other—I masturbated with doubled energy after each such incident. I felt overwhelming lust, I was constantly thinking about sex. I began to imagine that I was a victim of rape, that several men made love to me at the same time. Although nothing changed at home, I began to look at my father differently. I knew that I loved him like no one else. I was afraid of him, I felt disgust and lust, all at once. I was thirteen when Jehovah's Witnesses came to our house. Father began studying Bible with them. My brother and I listened. Although this religion demands that its followers change their way of life (it's supposed to be based on the rules imposed by Jehovah), father did not change his behavior. As for me, I was delighted with everything I heard. It was my hope. Father slowly lost his authority in my eyes. I knew that he behaved against Jehovah's principles. Nothing changed, however. I know that he was looking for a great romantic love, he had several affairs, but all of them ended. He continued to torment us. I think he hated Mother. They married because she had got pregnant, but he was mean for her and for us. He was a sadist. He did not get baptized. Apparently, he knew he wouldn't be able to change his life. But I began to regularly attend meetings of the Witnesses. One day at a meeting, an older brother asked, "Joanna, why don't you get baptized?" I was too young to tell him that I didn't feel ready. My father would probably kill me if I said what was happening at home. I regret that I didn't tell the brothers the truth about my home and about myself, about masturbation, they would have helped me. For sure. But I decided that since the older brother asked me that question, I had to be baptized. The moment he told me that, I got captivated. Captivated with Him. I felt that I loved Him. I got baptized at the earliest opportunity and didn't regret it. The more I learned the Bible, the stronger my faith became. At the same time, I got completely mad about sex. I still dreamed about rapes, I was ready to hurl myself into the arms of any boy who'd groove on me. I still masturbated many times during the day, although I knew how much Jehovah disapproved it. I should have talked to a sister from the congregation, but I didn't say anything. At that time a boy from my class started to appeal to me, the most aggressive, cold, and indifferent one. I started to dream about him. I knew the guys from the congregation, they were polite, cultured, the ones who kiss you on the hand. I met them, accompanied by a sister to supervise us, but even though we had a nice time, something else appealed to me—that boy and obsessive thoughts about sex and rape. We started to go out together. It wasn't great, he wasn't good to me. He blackmailed me that if I left him, he'd hang himself. He was malicious, but I still loved him madly. We started having sex. I knew that it wasn't right, that God didn't like it, that I was a harlot. I felt wonderful with him. He had unbelievable ideas. We made love in public places, in the elevator, in the park, etc., he liked it. Although I tried to tell him it was wrong, I agreed to it. I didn't want to lose him. I got pregnant. My "love" didn't feel ready for the role of a father. I aborted my pregnancy. I felt guilty. I told it to the brothers and sisters in the congregation. They didn't urge me to marry, but they sort of showed me that I was stuck in a sin. They met my boyfriend. We studied the Bible together. Having got to know him, they told me to rethink it, they said he was a difficult man. In retrospect, I think that he and my father were alike—he was also cold, self-interested, sadistic, got pleasure out of tormenting me. He could not talk to me for months. To my insistence, he'd only say "kiss my a . . . ," and yet he wouldn't let me go. I even tried to date with others. One of the "others" even beat my boyfriend, but I continued to be in this relationship. Studying the Bible, we knew that intercourse before marriage is a sin. We both promised that we would restrain ourselves from having sex. However, we broke this promise three times. I told the brothers and elders about this in the congregation. I was expelled. What was done was done. I had to legalize the relationship. We got married. There were many misunderstandings. My husband claimed that I could do nothing. I felt terrible. I actually couldn't do much. My father did everything at home. He said nobody was able to do anything as well as him. On the one hand, he forced us to work, on the other—he wouldn't let us. He said we were useless. If I made it to do something at home, I was looking for approval and acceptance from my father. I never had it, everything was done wrong. So I'm not surprised that I didn't have much idea about housekeeping. For example, I thought that washing windows is a man's job. My husband thought differently. I got married looking for a copy of Daddy.

Our son, Martin, was born. My husband persuaded me to leave C. The child suffered from celiac disease, and had excellent medical care here. I was afraid that in the village, in the middle of nowhere, there would be no such care, but I couldn't oppose my husband. Someone always had to boss me around. I wrote to the Witnesses that I had legalized the relationship. I was accepted again. We left to a small village near K. We weren't getting on well there. My husband began to drink unnoticed. He didn't help me at home. He forced me to have sex when I was tired the most. I tried to talk to him, I tried to convince him that if he helped me during the day, I'd have strength and desire at night. But the argument didn't speak to him. I felt that our marriage was falling apart. I decided to come back to C. with my son. We stayed at my parents'. Father just returned from the USA, where he had tried to start a new life for the last couple of years. He had money. Mother tried to persuade him to buy us a flat, but he didn't want to hear about it. He said we weren't worth it. Mother got ill. She was admitted to a detoxification ward by mistake. My brother used his contacts to put mother in a geriatric ward at a mental hospital. Dr. R. pulled her through that breakdown. She spent three months there. Immediately after she came back home, my father went to the same ward. They couldn't find the right drugs for him for a long time. They didn't cope with his aggression. He stayed half a year there. He came back changed.

My husband returned to the countryside. Parents bought me a room with a kitchen and I asked him to come back to me and start a new life. But he already had another woman, he didn't want to come back. I asked the Witnesses if it was possible that I wouldn't be with my husband. They said "Yes." Separation was possible, but not divorce. "You must learn to live without a man." It wasn't difficult. Sex with my husband made it repulsive to me. I thought, "I can live without my husband, I have God who's always with me, He'll always help me. There are also the brothers from the congregation, they won't leave me." And it was so. Together with my son, we were Jehovah's Witnesses, attended classes and meetings, we prayed together. My son learned very well. His teacher at school was an angel. She was an extremely tolerant person, and because she knew that I was bringing up my son alone, she tried to compensate him for the lack of his father and to bolster his confidence. In addition, he became friends with the owner of the pet shop, helped him in the store, fed animals and the like. He kept a turtle and fish at home. He cared for the aquarium himself. I met this man, I wanted to make sure that the friendship with him wasn't wrong for the boy. He turned out to be all right.

In January this year, I asked my husband to finally declare whether he'd come back to us or not. He came to C. and announced that he'd never come back. He was making a life with someone else now. It crushed me. I began to ask him not to leave me, otherwise I wanted him to kill me and the child too. He only said: "You're exaggerating." He didn't follow me completely. Then my ordeal began. I woke up one day and realized that God had left me. I tried to pray, but it was like praying to a brick wall. I tried . . . (here the patient begins to sob). Suddenly, I saw the truth! I'd never been a Jehovah's Witness, I was baptized in sin! It hit me that I'd always been in the hands of Satan. I heard his mocking laughter in my soul! Please, understand me well, in my soul! Satan is wiser and stronger than anyone—than you, than the ward head, than Mrs. P. He led me into a trap. He can do it. I'd always served him, not God. I still tried to pray. I begged: "Jehovah, let me at least kill myself! You let Judas, let me too!" But God didn't hear me! He wasn't with me. I prayed to a brick wall. I told the Witnesses about it. They didn't understand me, they said that God hadn't left me. But what could they know? God turned his face away from me! Anyway, everything suddenly changed around me. My son began to behave strangely. He started to buy dozens of notebooks or pens. He stopped caring for the fish, although he bought more and more of them. There was no room for them all in the aquarium, they were dying. He stopped eating, ran out barely dressed in the freezing cold, said he wanted to get pneumonia and die. He didn't eat anything at home but ice cream. He wanted to get cold and die. I asked a sister from the congregation to take care of him, maybe he would start eating with her children, but she told me that when he was with them, he just sat there and stared blankly at the television. I was indifferent to it in some way. I knew that my child, in-nocent as a lamb, must suffer, that he's fated to death, because he is my son. He stopped going to school. I knew it had to be so. I felt sorry for him, I couldn't stand his sufferings, but he was under the power of Satan. He asked, "Mommy, why aren't we Jehovah's Witnesses anymore?" Though, at the end of the first grade, he wrote in his notebook that serving Jehovah, God, is the most important thing. So I saw that the child was experiencing the same as me. I thought we were stigmatized only because I'm my father's daughter. When Mother was pregnant with my brother, Father put poison in front of them both, told her to take it, and he intended to kill himself too. They didn't do it, but he was also under the power of Satan. My son bought toy guns at that time, put them to his temple and asked me to buy a real weapon, kill him first, then myself. I knew I had to do that. I started to go to the market in search of a weapon, but Satan made me unable to buy it. And I wasn't able to kill my child in any other way. Of course it was Satan's fault, all my friends have weapons, only I don't. How was I supposed to kill my son? I'd have had to tighten a noose around his neck or smother him. I couldn't do that! To carry your baby in you for months, to nurse it, and then kill it? I was already guilty of one murder, I killed someone, I had an abortion! Finally, a psychologist from his school visited us, but my son ran away. Then he only repeated that he didn't want to live. I wrote a letter to his teacher. I explained that although we were Jehovah's Witnesses, we were now under the power of Satan. My son barely went to school at that time. He forgot how to write. He just couldn't. The teacher informed his father. In June this year, he came to us and took our son with him. He said he'd look after him. The child didn't oppose him, but he called me a pig, and his father a dick. He shouted, "Kill me! I don't want to live, it's all because of you!" But he didn't say anything to his father, he went with him. Sometimes he calls me, supervised by his father, or writes and asks about his turtle, but I poured the fish out, I was too weak to keep them. I stopped bathing, I wanted to starve myself, but I couldn't eat nothing. So I decided to eat only bread with margarine, nothing more. I lost over ten kilos. Maybe I'll die more slowly this way, but I eventually will. I started to look for death. I walked on the roofs, I wanted to jump, but I wasn't allowed. I wanted to poison myself, but failed. I know why. Satan tells me sneeringly, "Oh no, dear, you won't die so easily." So how will I die? Will they cut me into slices, will I have to eat human feces, will they burn me with fire or will they make me drown slowly? What is the worst death Satan is preparing for me? I will not die so easily, I know. Nothing or no one will help me, and God turned away from me. I was baptized in sin, so I was never a Jehovah's Witness, I only thought so. I've served Satan all the time. I can compare my situation only to the one of Eve in Paradise—she didn't want to leave it either, but Satan laid a snare for her. And now he's laying one for me. The brothers come and say that I'm not expelled, but I'm begging them to stop coming here, because something bad could happen to them, because of me. I'm afraid anyone who contacts me is stigmatized. I know there's no help for me. Mother forced me to go to the doctor. But I didn't even get my prescriptions filled. I know that even a bucket of drugs won't help me. I did it for my mother, because father said I was finishing her off. I had to listen to him. But I know there's no help for me. Doctor Z. doesn't know that everything is an ambush and Satan's snares. Why mustn't I die?! Why doesn't Jehovah have mercy? How will I die?! And he's just laughing. He's more powerful than anyone and anything.

Joanna's story begins with the father figure and ends with the words "father," "Jehovah," and "Satan." We can consider this symbolic frame as the basis for interpretation. The family life events and religion interconnect within this frame. Let us try to follow the clearest nodal points of both themes. Joanna's father, apart from his episodes of depression (the patient mentioned it during anamnesis), showed evident psychopathic features, he probably suffered from anankastic personality disorder ("he was crazy about cleaning," "he was constantly cleaning something").[7] He manipulated his family members, humiliated and abused them, he did not refrain from sexually abusing his daughter. Joanna says much about her father, which is certainly not a coincidence, but indicates that her conscious psyche is occupied with him to a large extent. Joanna talks very little about her mother, she mainly says that she was the father's victim. This was the reason why she hated the mother, which is quite a typical reaction of a child who hates a parent for being weak (fights at home are threatening for the child, and the parent, who does not withstand, is perceived as complicit in the situation).

Joanna's attitude to her father is very important for the understanding of the course of her disease and the character of her religiousness. It was very ambivalent. Her first (or the first related to her father's violence) memory is the situation built up of emotional conflicts: the father feeds her and at the same time beats her mother. And if he beats the mother, he certainly produces a sense of danger in the child. He is both a caretaker and an aggressor. The first memories of childhood, even if they were only memory illusions, can express the patient's basic psychological complexes in a vivid way. They are representations of mental structures that involve a lot of energy, and in a subconscious way affect experiencing and behavior. We can say they are unconscious fantasies. Joanna's first memory may express such an unconscious fantasy: a caretaker must also be a persecutor. This mental script tells her later to choose this and not another partner, it will also affect her image of God.

Joanna's ambivalence increased enormously and became fixed when the father began to sexually abuse her. Joanna felt strong sexual impulses since early childhood, she began to masturbate very early. Masturbation was a way to relax, find peace and a sense of security among the tensions that prevailed at home. When her father started to sexually abuse her, he filled her with disgust, but on the other hand she became more and more aroused, and masturbation probably gave her even more pleasure. It is hard to imagine the intensity of the conflicting emotions that must be experienced by a girl who is at the threshold of puberty and is sexually abused by her father. One can say without hesitation that it is impossible to extricate oneself from such a situation and remain mentally healthy.

Joanna's psyche had to deal with this multitude of affect. Despite the fact that she was constantly afraid of her father and felt disgusted with him, she could not negate him. On the contrary, she began to "love him like no one else." She did not want to lose the positive image of the father, so to maintain the relationship with him, she developed a sufficiently strong reaction opposite to the emotions and tendencies (disgust and fear) that crushed this relationship. In this way, as a result of the conversion of negative feelings to their opposite, her great "love" to her father emerged. Her sexual desire and satisfaction obtained as a result of masturbation played a significant role in the formation of this feeling. When Joanna became interested in religion, when she learned about God Jehovah, her father "slowly lost his authority." [8]

We cannot, based on the text we have, discover all the motivational factors that made her react so strongly to religious themes and become involved in them so much. Perhaps one of the factors was the possibility of displacing a part of the affect she had for her father onto another object. Onto the "father" who is much more perfect and gives more protection. The God of Jehovah's Witnesses seems to have a stronger paternal component than the Catholic God—He is the only one, He has neither a Son nor a Spirit "next to" Him. There is also no Marian cult in this religion, and let us remember that Joanna hated her mother.

Note some similarity in the form of her talking about how she realized the love for her father ("I began to look at my father differently. I knew that I loved him like no one else") and about the "captivation" she experienced later, feeling that she loved God ("I got captivated. Captivated with Him. I felt that I loved Him"). In both cases there is a moment of sudden change. Also, the moment she learned about Jehovah, her father lost in significance.

Because of religion, Joanna partly abandoned her father on the emotional level, but the drive impulses aroused during sexual intercourse with him exploded with even greater force ("The more I learned the Bible, the stronger my faith became. At the same time, I got completely mad about sex"). She was ready to hurl herself into the arms of any boy who would show her some warmth and interest. Joanna began to separate herself and her needs more and more from the father figure. At this moment, there are three main objects in whom she invested feelings: the father, Jehovah, and a potential boyfriend. Joanna, withdrawing some libido from the father figure, gained additional energy to get involved emotionally outside her family. Here, Joanna's sexuality could become even more intense because she was no longer stopped by the feeling of disgust associated with it. Although she freed her sexuality from the father figure—which was positive from the developmental point of view—Joanna remained dependent and did not lose her emotional contact with the "father." The father, in whom she now invested the sensitive elements of her emotional life, became Jehovah. In a row, the object onto which she transferred her sexual expectations was her boyfriend, then her husband. However, both of them took over the indestructible heritage of the relationship with her biological father.

Joanna realized how much the one she chose was like her father. And how their relationship reminded her of the relationship with him. She was not aware, however, that also God that she experienced in herself, slowly took on the characteristics of the father. The relationship with her husband made her suffer, but she could not live in another one. Her inner structure, shaped in childhood, did not allow her to live in a different way or with anyone else. The strength of the emotional stigma of childhood translated into a string of unsound decisions and failures, conditioned by the repetition compulsion.

When her husband declared that he would never come back to her (though they had not been together for a long time), Joanna broke down. Then she lost the ability to cope with her life and her illness manifested itself. Her husband's declaration influenced her so badly that she begged him to kill her and the child. Regardless of whether it was a real request or just a dramatic expression of distress, it shows how desperate she was. It was just after her husband's declaration that she woke up one day and felt that God had left her. She tried to pray, but she felt that her prayers were ignored, that she was praying "to a brick wall" because there was no longer any person who would be sensitive to her fate. Then, in Joanna's life, the figure of Satan appeared. Joanna felt that she had always served Satan, not God. The relative stabilization of her life collapsed. The problems with her son grew, and he began to show the symptoms of obsessive-compulsive disorder (buying notebooks and pens), so similar to those of his grandfather. Her sense of guilt increased, which became one of the basic factors determining the further course of Joanna's suffering. It involved the memory of the aborted pregnancy, her father's reproaches ("I did it for my mother, because Father said I was finishing her off"). It also had an unconscious current that cannot be accurately analyzed based on the available material, but its probable components can be named.

Joanna's husband was a substitute for her father, and the images of both men in her psyche overlapped. Losing her husband, she in a way lost the father, which meant that her relatively stable relationship with his image was destroyed. In this way, the "father" turned away from her, left her, and thus doomed her to the monstrous guilt of the past. Joanna felt the abandonment and burden of guilt in the most intense manner. She experienced them in relation to the image of God (onto which the libidinal cathexis was transferred from the representation of her father), and expressed them in the words: "God turned his face away from me!"

As for the question of Satan, Joanna seems to link his activities with her father. Referring to the negative influence of Satan on her son and her life, she at the same time utters the significant words: "I thought we were stigmatized only because I'm my father's daughter." Note that Satan harms Joanna on the one hand, but he does not let her die and stands in the way of killing her son on the other. Even if she explains it as part of his plan to make her die a more horrible death, it must be understood as protection. We need to interpret this type of fantasy in its basic form, so as Satan-who-protects. Here, we return to Joanna's original ambivalence towards her father, which is apparent in her memory of the father who is feeding her and is threatening at the same time.[9] So Satan is modeled after the father. He appears when Joanna has no one with her, and he is the only figure who can bring something positive into her life (the protective aspect). This is analogous to the situation of a child who usually prefers a relationship with a bad object to the lack of relationship.

Finally, note the grammatical ambiguity (amphiboly) in the last sentences. Who is laughing? Satan or Jehovah? Perhaps this is not a simple error, but another reference to the close relation between the most important figures in Joanna's life.

## NOTES

1. Freud acknowledged the importance of both parents in the formation of religiousness, but he attributed different functions to them. According to him, the mother played the role only in relation to the religion of nature and the father was to play the central role in creating the image of God in monotheistic religions. Some of his successors had a different point of view, stressing the function of the mother or parental couple as a whole (Rizzuto 1990). Also, academic psychology research indicates that the mother figure plays a significant role in shaping the individual image of God (see Wulff 1999, 272).

2. "Transference neurosis" is a condition in which most of the patient's pathological reactions are directed towards the figure of the therapist. As a result of the positive development of the therapy, after a longer period of its duration, there is a specific transformation of neurosis in the clinical sense into transference neurosis (Laplanche and Pontalis 2006, 462–63). Earlier, there are more rambling transference reactions (transference is an unconscious directing of anxiety, associations, needs, and pathological reactions formed in early childhood to the analyst).

3. A term coined by Jung—an archetypal vision of a personified or embodied supernatural power (god, hero, priest).

4. The compulsion to repeat (repetition compulsion) is an unconscious motivational process that causes the person to actively expose himself to distressing situations, thereby repeating his previous traumatic experiences. He does not realize that the current events have a prototype, but considers them as new and determined only by the circumstances of the moment (see Laplanche and Pontalis 2006, 78–80).

5. Transactional analysis refers to three *ego* states: the Parent, Adult, and Child state. Our *ego* alters the state depending on the nature of the interpersonal relationship—for example, it will use one of them when talking to the head director, and a different one when meeting an invalid asking for help.

6. According to *ICD-10* (*International Statistical Classification of Diseases and Related Health Problems*), schizoaffective disorder is a mental disorder characterized by schizophrenia-like symptoms as well as affective disorder symptoms (depression, mania), with both types of symptoms reaching similar intensity.

7. Anankastic personality disorder, according to *ICD-10*, is characterized, inter alia, by pedantry, perfectionism and extreme orderliness (in a broad sense). In this case *DSM-5* refers to obsessive-compulsive personality disorder.

8. According to Jehovah's Witnesses, "Jehovah" is the "true name of God." This word (*Jehovah*) was created by filling the Hebrew tetragrammaton of JHWH with the vowels of the word *Adonai* ("Lord"), which the Jews use to describe God (Langkammer 1993, 83).

9. According to Freud, emotional ambivalence is by nature related to the father figure (Freud 1961a). That is why he is a prototype of both God and Satan. In the history of religion, the image of deity (e.g., Yahweh)—based on the image of father—full of contradictions, has been divided into a good and evil figure (God and the devil).

*Chapter Four*

# Anorexia Nervosa: A Pathological Attempt at Deification

## AN ASTONISHING DISEASE

In psychiatry, it is possible to diagnose anorexia in a man (these are rare cases—it is estimated that the ratio of men to women suffering from the disorder is approximately 1:10), however, I consider "male anorexia" to be a different disorder, and when I speak of anorexia, I mean the problem that concerns women. I have observed the compact and repetitive psychopathological structure described here only in women. It is not just a refusal to eat, but it contains a whole set of unconscious motives. Anorexia, as I describe it, is a disease of women due to, among other things, physiological differences between the sexes—a dieting man would not be able to achieve so many changes of such great meaning in life. To put it simply, one can say that a man who slims changes "quantitatively," while a woman who slims to extremes changes "qualitatively." For example, ovulation stops abruptly as a result of starvation, while sperm production falls gradually. A slimming anorexic to a certain extent "ceases to be a woman" at the physical level, because she becomes incapable of the basic sexual function, that is, reproduction. That is why "ordinary slimming" can become a tool for relieving internal conflicts, a peculiar "way of life."

Anorexia nervosa confronts us with the issue of the incomprehensible connections between the mind and the body, and tests the colloquial and commonsense understanding of human behavior. One of the first thoughts that almost always come to people confronted with this illness is the impatient question: "Why doesn't she just start eating?" We do not understand why a girl whose health and life are in danger cannot eat normally. We do not realize the extreme intensity of her anxiety about weight gain, about food, or about the act of eating. Asking the patient herself rarely changes anything, as she often gives the most banal reasons for her state, such as her desire to "get slimmer." The repeating patterns of anorexic patients' behaviors and views are astonishing. The disorder forms a compact psychological structure, the shape of which consists of certain behaviors, thoughts, emotions, a specific style of entering into relationships, and given elements of the patient's family system.

## THE ISOLATED *EGO*, A REJECTION OF THE BODY

We can understand anorexia as an attempt to separate the *ego* from the factors that influence it, an attempt to strengthen and free it; an attempt to create an isolated *ego*. One of the fundamental factors limiting the feeling of power of the *ego* is the body. It functions in a significant measure independently of the will and consciousness; it also has its own rights and needs. The anorexic rejects the awkward body in order to become a self-contained, self-sufficient *ego*.

The image of the isolated *ego* is the basis of what the anorexic thinks and does. This is an archetype, a mental teleological structure.[1] It models the girl's psyche and draws her towards the model that is physically out of reach. The anorexic, overwhelmed by such an image, wants to reject everything that could restrict her, to be free and independent of the drives and everything that is associated with the functions of the body. This is the most important, albeit to varying degrees conscious, goal of every anorexic. She identifies with her own *ego*, and wants it to represent her entire person. The remaining spheres, that include emotions and drives independent of the *ego*, are repulsed from the sphere of her identity.[2]

Of course, the anorexic cannot really reject her own body and become the self-contained *ego*. So she rejects the body which she cannot control, and accepts only the one she creates herself. Initially, the image of the body that she creates fits the socially preferred standard more and more (slim figure), but after a short time, it becomes completely different. Usually, the anorexic is not concerned by this, and if so, the inner forces turn out to be stronger than her doubts. They may even be so strong as to lead the sick woman to death. This is the unquestionable evidence that the problem of anorexia is not limited to the impact of the "model image," but as a matter of fact it does not have much in common with it. The image of a slim female body is actually just a trigger element, which opens the way to deeper motivating factors. It also becomes a part of secondary rationalization of the motives that the sufferer is not aware of.

The anorexic starts to live according to the emerging, archetypal image, as it acts as an attractor modelling the shape of her life within the defined limits. Anorexia is an attempt to really achieve the archetypal features which philosophy, and even more so theology, attributes to a special being, namely the "absolute *ego*," God. The image of the isolated *ego* covers at least the essential points of the visions of the Absolute, Wholeness, or God. These ideas are either interchangeable with the image of the pure *ego* or have its constitutive characteristics. The fact that various concepts of the "absolute *ego*" are constantly formed within philosophy and theology indicates that they lie in the very structure of the mind. The archetypal structure of the absolute *ego* is responsible both for the creation of such visions as well as for the course of anorexia.

## THE STRUCTURE OF THE ARCHETYPAL ISOLATED *EGO*

The speculation of St. Thomas Aquinas is one of the most prototypical philosophical visions of God. St. Thomas's idea of God presents Him as completely "simple," which means He is not a "body," He is "in no way composite," He is invariable (Thomas Aquinas 1999, 139). Let us have a closer look at the premises of divine simplicity, namely "the identity of God and His essence." This speculation, rooted in the philosophy of Aristotle, constantly recurs in the later history of theology when it refers to God. St. Thomas writes:

> God is the same as His essence or nature. To understand this, it must be noted that in things composed of matter and form, the nature or essence must differ from the *suppositum*, for the essence or nature includes only what falls within the definition of the species; as humanity includes all that falls within the definition of man, for it is by this that man is man, and it is this that humanity signifies that, namely, whereby man is man. Now individual matter, with all the individuating accidents, does not fall within the definition of the species. For this particular flesh, these bones, this blackness or whiteness, etc., do not fall within the definition of a man. Therefore this flesh, these bones, and the accidental qualities designating this particular matter, are not included in humanity; and yet they are included in the reality which is a man. Hence, the reality which is a man has something in it that humanity does not have. Consequently, humanity and a man are not wholly identical, but humanity is taken to mean the formal part of a man, because the principles whereby a thing is defined function as the formal constituent in relation to the individuating matter. (Thomas Aquinas 1999, 133)

I would like to assure those who found the above scholastic deliberations boring that it addresses the aspects of our mental functioning. I believe that this vision is the result of projection of certain internal states and their rationalization. The vision, therefore, stems from a specific self-reflection.

For centuries, philosophers have discussed the "necessary being" and "contingent beings," the "essence" of things and their "existence" different from that "essence." In fact, it was the search for what really *is*. Because if something develops, it never truly exists. It constantly leaves behind that which it has just been. And it is not yet that which it soon will be. In man, his "existence" is different from his "essence," as that who and what he is does not explain at all or justify his existence. Man does not own himself for himself, he was not the one who created him and is not the one who maintains his existence (he does not, for example, support physiological changes in his body with a constant act of will; they happen irrespective of his will and consciousness). So the discussed philosophical reflection was built on the observation that it is possible to distinguish as if two spheres in man, one of which would be something more defined, existing, or "my own," and the other one less so. This splitting—depending on the aspect that was taken into account—was referred to as a division into the "soul" and "body," "form" and "matter," "nature" and "subject," "necessity" and "contingency," "act" and "potency."[3] Perceiving the sphere of "perfection" must have resulted from the self-reflection on the structure of mind, consciousness, or our *ego* (understood mainly as "the observing *ego*" not confounded in conflicts).[4] The distinction of the other area resulted from the observation of one's dependence on the body that is not fully controllable. From the psychological point of view, we can speak of the split between the *ego* and the drives, between the conscious and volitional and the involuntary, of the split between the sphere of control and the uncontrollable sphere, between the *coiled-up* area and the area in *participation*.

Man could not free himself from this tormenting division. The randomness and defectiveness of life disappeared only in the idea of God, who, as a "simple" being, was a justification for Himself. He did not have any "autonomous" elements that are not fully controllable (like the body, the unconscious). St. Thomas's God is "a being in action," fully realized, which means that He already is everything He can be. This corresponds to His immateriality, as matter always has a certain potential, and it can become something different from what it is at the moment. Being immaterial, He is also indivisible, and thus constant. In all of Thomas's speculation, immateriality, constancy, realization, unity, and perfection intertwine. In earlier concepts, similar features were attributed to the "being," to this what really is, that was treated as partially sacred. Before St. Thomas, an earlier philosopher, Melissus of Samos, said that the being:

> must not have body; but if it had thickness, it would have parts, and no longer be one. (quoted in Quarantotto 2018, 76)

Similarly, Plato constructed his idea of the soul, which he considered to be timeless, and thus the only valuable, part of man. The body was just its residence, or rather a cage that does not allow the fullness of humanity to be revealed. In *Phaedo*, he wrote:

> And thought is best when the mind is gathered into herself and none of these things trouble her—neither sounds nor sights nor pain nor any pleasure,—when she has as little as possible to do with the body, and has no bodily sense or feeling, but is aspiring after being? (Plato 1993, 63)

## THE ARCHETYPE OF THE ISOLATED *EGO* IN ANOREXIA

The anorexic wishes to be human without the flawed sphere of "contingency" or "matter." She wants to be "herself," and dispose of everything of which she cannot say with certainty, "This is me." In the words of the Eleatic philosophy of Melissus: the anorexic wants to be "one," to have no "thickness." The body, however, stands in the way of achieving it. And so do the related drives, such as the hunger drive. Drives, just like the body, are something that defy the decisions of the *ego*. They can "hit" the *ego*, and collide with the environment. The anorexic fears this, so she "attracts" back to her everything that does not "fit," and that might lead to an uncontrolled contact with the world (anorexics often react adversely to accidental contacts, for example they are disproportionately afraid to touch someone on the bus and get irritated when somebody accidentally jostles them). She achieves this through minimizing her drive activity (fast) and her own bodily dimensions. Thanks to this, she—symbolically and literally—reduces the surface of her contact with the world.

According to the stoics, people should only worry about what they can influence and leave the rest. Marcus Aurelius wrote:

> You are composed of three things: body, breath, and mind. The first two belong to you in so far as you need to take care of them, but only the third is yours in the proper sense. So if you detach from yourself, that is, from your own mind whatever other people do or say or whatever you yourself have done or said, and all the anticipations of the future that disturb you and all the extraneous involuntary aspects of the body that envelops you [. . .] and if you make yourself, in the words of Empedocles, 'a well-rounded sphere, rejoicing in its circular solitude' [. . .] then you will be able to live out the time that is left until you die in a manner that is free of upset and good-natured, at peace with your own divine spirit [daímōn]. (Marcus Aurelius 2018, 56)

Only the mind is absolutely ours and the anorexic wants to reduce herself to it. However, she does not leave the rest of herself and her life to its own course. To create a "sphere" of herself, she actively cuts off the rest of her person. The anorexic wants to be the "mind" or "soul." Her body, and above all one of its components—"fat"—makes achieving this goal impossible. She has a vision of "fat" that lives a life of its own, and takes her away from herself. While a healthy person is not afraid of losing his identity due to having a body, the anorexic feels that her essence (soul, the *ego*) is constantly endangered by it. For the anorexic her bones and skin are like a "form" (or "spirit"), while fat is matter.

Extreme weight loss also allows the anorexic to avoid assessment. It is another form of "disappearing" from the field of interpersonal interactions, and thus another way to fully own herself. Young girls mature differently than young boys—their development involves a greater qualitative change (menstruation, significant change in body shape), so when they enter the adult life, accepting the body and its functions requires special effort. On the social level, a woman as a person is assessed much more based on her appearance. A woman enters men's field of perception, marked with eroticism and evaluation, and it is here that she must establish her identity. The anorexic, however, remains as if in the phase of potentiality, suspended between all possible choices. She has not yet adopted any socially recognized identity, and cannot be defined or judged.

One of the patients explained to me, "It all started with my legs." Her family joked about how thin they were. And so the girl decided, paradoxically, to make them even thinner, to "change their shape." For what purpose? In a certain sense, legs which have been slimmed to the extreme evade all judgment, as they become simply an example of the standard anatomy of lower limbs. Thus, the patient "regained" her legs only for herself, and made it impossible for the environment to assess them. Stopping the independent development of her body, she reached a state similar to St. Thomas's "being in the act," where everything that can happen is already there, and is fully internalized, controllable (belongs to the "essence").

Anorexics very often feel anxiety and resistance when someone tells them that they "look better," or that they have a "round face" and the like (in a situation, for example, where the girl started to bend to the social pressure and fight her eating disorder). The anorexic starts to panic, feels "fat," and "horrible." With the comments, she stops controlling the environment's opinion, and ceases to be "self-referential." Her body starts to "live its own life," and becomes a form of public property. In her eyes, the anorexic begins to lose the status of being spontaneous, having all of her for her own. When she gains weight, she feels that everyone can see something else in her, and she has no control over it. This is an important moment. Now she feels as if somebody else could take a piece of her for themselves.[5]

The girl's body, her exterior, starts to take on its own individual properties, while she—conversely—begins to feel that she is one of the many, a "grey person." Earlier, she was given a lot of attention, and that interest was pleasant and important to her. She had the impression that it touched her essence, and at the same time only this that she knew and controlled. The narcissistic aspect of anorexia is a kind of aversion to be "just a person" ("a grey person," "one of the many," "an ordinary person").

The anorexic wishes to be the sole creator of her own life, and is irritated by any form of submission to objective conditions (Margaret, twenty-seven years old: "I was terribly obsessed with the thought that couldn't create myself out of nothing, that I could only reduce myself to these bones. I realized that I wouldn't create myself fully, it was such an unpleasant feeling"). The desired, "pure" *ego* of the anorexic wants to be subjected only to the will, independent of everything which is not the *ego*. The anorexic does not want to acknowledge the impact of time, the passage of which is mostly manifested in the body. Through her actions, she attains imaginary freedom of time, as the natural indicators of its passing, such as bodily changes or menstruation occurring in mature women, disappear.

The anorexic desires what is unchangeable. However, her body—as in every human—is subjected to the physiological process resulting from the passage of time. A static state is impossible. That is why she tries, through slimming, to change the course of development processes, even reverse the arrow of time. Because only when the slimming process constantly progresses, her control over the reality-body is relatively maintained. That is why anorexics are usually unsatisfied with what they have already achieved. They continually want less. Unable to achieve immutability, they try to replace the normal physiological process with the regressive one, the divergent sequence—with the convergent one, the uncertain future of the developing organism—with the imaginary safety of involution.

## THE STRUCTURE OF THE *SELF*

Eating points to our dependence on the world and proves that we are not self-sufficient. The overwhelming sensation of hunger makes us aware of it. This lack of autonomy and dependence on the drive is a source of anxiety that the anorexic tries to deny. Anorexics are often extremely critical about manifestations of human drives and corporeality, and criticize other's eating-related behaviors (Margaret: "I couldn't look at people eating, because it seemed so savage to me . . . as if they had no control over the activity"; "I perceived a day as a larger continuity. I wouldn't expect any presents from my day like lessening the tension, having a snack. I saw that other people had such a moment in their day, such a crisis—at noon for example—that they wanted something for themselves: 'OK, we're working and working, studying and studying, let's have some me-time now.' And this most often meant eating. It evoked such revulsion or loathing in me that they go after it!"). Being so critical, anorexics also constantly sense the threat of bulimia (association expressed by Isabella, sixteen years old: "a cracking dam and water flooding everything"), as a compensative response of the drive aspect of the organism. Because the rejected sphere becomes darker and darker, and its manifestations are more and more impulsive, the anorexic turns eating meals into a peculiar ceremony, which, as in obsessive-compulsive disorder, is to restrict the spontaneous drive activity (Alice, twenty-one years old: "Everything must be served properly, I always must have my dinner on my plate. I can't eat when something is done differently"). Although the anorexic refuses to take food, she cannot detach herself from matters related to eating. Quite the opposite, she is obsessively addicted to them. They fill her mind and determine her behaviors. She takes over the control of the kitchen and prepares meals for the family. And paying unusual attention to food caloric values, besides its practical significance, is to rationalize the drives that fill her. Usually, the anorexic feels overwhelmingly forced to cook meals, portion them, serve to other family members, and watch their behavior in the kitchen or attitude towards food. This may be a source of numerous family conflicts because the sufferer reacts impulsively to any objections of the household members to her dictating what and when they should eat. If she is removed from the kitchen, she perceives it as a threat (Patricia, twenty years old: "As if they had taken the last field I was good at") and usually reacts with an anxiety attack combined with a burst of anger and grievance. What happens here?

The anorexic, within the culinary sphere, fulfils and manifests a part of her personality. If removed from the kitchen, she feels that her own identity is endangered. This results from her specific mental structure. She *coils up* her *ego* because in her psyche she perceives fields with no unified boundaries. The realms that remain in *participation* can be controlled only through external activities, such as preparing meals. The anorexic's behaviors towards food do not follow the normal pattern of "person/object," but are far more complex. The "person" is "less" or differently separated here. In the case of anorexia, the following working scheme may be suggested: "*me/not-me*," where *not-me* would include the body, the sphere of emotions and drives, as well as the spectrum of matters related to the eating process. Therefore, on the one hand, for the anorexic, her body and emotions are more "external" than for a healthy person; on the other hand, food, eating activities and processes become in a way "psychisized." Figuratively speaking: the anorexic rejects her body and emotions, pushes them to the "external" sphere, where they "mix" with the nourishment issues, food, meals, dietetics, etc., and return to her in this new form.[6]

It happens that the anorexic sufferer tends to collect stashes of food around the house. These may be sweets, fruit, and similar delicacies. If a stash is discovered and taken away, the anorexic loses her temper. One of the patients told me that she "got hysterical" when she noticed that the sweets she had hidden were gone. She hid these delicacies in order to eat them later. But usually she either had to throw them away or she gave them to a household member after a few days. It was important to her, however, that they were her secret possession for some time. Trying to capture the psychological meanings that occur here, we must say that the anorexic perceives these things as much more than mere possessions; she experiences them as a part of herself (*participation*). They are a substitute for the part of personality she has rejected.[7]

## FAMILY—MOTHER—PREGNANCY—FOOD

The anorexic strives for independence and freedom, as she feels she is entangled in the family system. She wants independence to avoid further problems, including those that may result from being a woman in the family. In this aspect, anorexia is the issue of sexual maturation of the young girl and is related to the Oedipal situation.[8] Within the family system, there are a number of pressure points, which the future anorexic perceives consciously and unconsciously, and which direct her life towards constricting her own development. The anorexic wishes to remain "neutral," to remain a child, she does not want to cause conflicts by her maturing and becoming a woman. The relationship with the mother is strongly characterized by ambivalence. On the one hand, the girl identifies with the mother, and strives for separation from her on the other. She may be strongly attached to the mother and adopt the role of her guardian, and at the same time, in the face of such an embarrassing attachment, more or less conscious anger with the mother occurs. The anorexic cannot separate herself from the mother because, among other reasons, she does not feel she has a strong father. She is afraid she will be the second woman next to her mother, because she perceives femininity in her family as pervasive and frightening. The anorexic feels that her individuality is threatened by the mother and at the same time is afraid to be separated from her, because a part of her personality exists and constitutes itself within this relationship. She is afraid that if she breaks this peculiar relationship, she will not be able to incorporate this "part" into herself. This shows clearly that anorexia is an identity crisis. Regarding the relationship with the mother, the anorexic may for instance feel forced to compare the amount of food she consumes to that eaten by her mother. This way, she tries to control the mother and keep a specific distance from her at the same time (if she eats less, she is distinctly "different" from the mother).

We may say that the mother seems "numinous" to the anorexic; she is dangerous and unpredictable. Refusal to take food compensates for such dependence on the mother, because the daughter now rejects what was the most desired thing throughout her infancy and what connected her to the mother most. Food is the mother's gift and message. During the infancy period, it informs of care, safety, and acceptance. Later on, serving and having meals may, however, become a kind of substitutive communication or even a communication barrier. In such a case, the family concentrates on the times of meals and the eating-related issues. Eating becomes a connector that consolidates the family, who would, otherwise, face a threat of internal conflicts and divisions. For example, a family meal introduces an element of unity because all individual family members function within a similar psychological and physiological modality determined by a universal biological rhythm. In simpler terms: tastes are more universal than views and approaches. Preparing and serving meals allows one to hide negative emotions and to avoid unsolved problems under the cover of friendly and rational actions (Margaret: "Mother could only feed me, she never noticed a woman inside me, nor wanted me to be one").

The fact that anorexia affects only women also results from the inseparable relation between eating and reproduction. Note that only a woman faces a situation where she is the food for another person: the fetus feeds on the substances circulating in the mother's blood, and the infant drinks the milk produced by her body. Both these situations are in fact examples of consuming the woman. The organism must secure itself from potential negative effects by increasing the fat tissue, and the woman herself must be on a proper diet throughout the pregnancy. The evolution theory and embryology prove that nature provides the best protection for the descendant; the pregnant woman's body is thus subordinated to the fetus's needs to a large extent. It has various psychological consequences. Since the woman feeds the child with a product of her own body and is—if one can say so—at risk of being "eaten" by the child, her attitude towards eating and food must be different than in men.

Let us look from the perspective of cultural patterns. "Femininity" is associated with carnality, feeding, passivity, periodicity, and dependence. It is characteristic that the anorexic functions as if she wanted to transcend the above elements. She seems to be directed towards archetypally understood "masculinity," expressed in rationality, activity, independence, and spirituality. The perfectionism typical of anorexics, unaccepting the undetermined, and over-rationalization (Alice: "It annoys me how my mother goes from one topic to the next; for me, a conversation needs to have a thesis and arguments, then I can accept the conclusion"; Margaret: "In anorexia, I had a lot more intellectual balance") are manifestations of the fixation on the *ego* (the *ego*, together with the subjected intellect, creates plans, patterns, classifications, and any order in the perceived world), and, at the same time, archetypally masculine elements.

Anorexia is also an attempt to remain, in some aspects, a child (Agatha, fourteen years old: "I'd like to be that child again, without all these problems, a child who read the Bible every day"), whose image is associated with freedom, beginning, and potentiality (though in many respects—for example, as being devoid of spontaneity and excessively controlling herself—the anorexic is the opposite of childness).

But the specific model of anorexia also consists of the image of an "elder," a person with a distanced approach to manifestations of life (Margaret: "There was a moment when I grabbed myself in the hands of this anorexic functioning that, when other girls went to get something to eat, I'd feel such peace as of a child and an old person. It suited me a lot. I always thought there was something vulgar about growing up"). It will not be difficult to demonstrate the common part of the above-mentioned modalities of life ("male," "elder," "child"). Men are commonly recognized as "eternal children" with their "relaxed" approach to life, while the elderly do not get involved in some aspects of it. All these dynamics—including what I have defined as "stopping" or "reversing" time—stem from the desire to escape femininity and the related factors that determine life. The anorexic cannot accept such limitations of freedom of the *ego* as the absolute repeatability of the menstrual cycle, and the potential enslavement by pregnancy. The body is a threat to her, as it can become, to a great extent, dependent on the supraindividual process of nature, the birthing process.

## SPIRITUALITY AND ENSLAVEMENT OF ANOREXICS

The issue of eating food was not neglected by any religion. Fasting, sacred feasts, prohibitions, and orders imposed on the culinary sphere serve as the regulators of life that occur in many religions. They are also symbols that express man's attitude towards the *sacrum*. It cannot omit the eating aspect, which, after all, shows our lack of autonomy the most.

In psychotherapy, not only in the case of anorexics, we observe that episodes of refusing to eat are a way to obtain emotional independence, to eliminate the "hunger for feelings." During therapy, the patient may have moments when she refrains from eating, as the need for dependence, that was formed in her childhood and is reconstructed in her relationship with the therapist, starts to scare her. This is a way to regain her self-sufficiency, a state of narcissistic fulfilment. Sometimes such symptoms occur in neurotic depression—the patient wishes to avoid contacts with people and reality, even if it is only in the form of food. These symptoms express her pursuing the image of God, who does not hunger for nor desire anything, being fulfilled in himself. Abstaining from eating, along with the feeling of lack of satiety, becomes for the anorexic a peculiar core, around which her sense of identity concentrates. We all know the feeling when we are sated after a meal—we become ponderous, as if we were melting in an armchair and in the world. The anorexic feels that she cannot allow herself to satisfy her hunger normally because it could destroy her psychic cohesion, crushing the identity to which she holds on with such an effort. Therefore, she chooses lack of satiability that causes a feeling of greater compactness.[9] Tertullian, using the language of theology, expresses the same, writing:

> Denying oneself food and drink leads to such a significant distinction. Man becomes a member of the household of God. The image is combined with the original. Because the Eternal—as testified through Isaiah the prophet—never feels hungry, there will come a time when man, like his God, will live as Him—without food. (Tertullian 2007, 106)

The God of the theologians is basically identical with the vision of the archetype of the isolated *ego* or the model of the Jungian model of *Self* (see Jung 1995, 186–88).[10] The images of Wholeness, the Absolute, or God—as I have tried to show it—correlate with the forces that really act in the human mind. They are not only passive products of the intellect, but actively affect behavior. They are present in our lives, even if we do not go to church and do not engage in philosophical deliberations. The anorexic's *ego* is attracted to this pattern associated with the image of psychological wholeness. In the first stage of slimming, when the organism has not been emaciated by physiological disorders yet, quite oppositely, has gained some new deposits of energy, anorexics feel their freedom and independence, which may border with a manic sense of omnipotence. The *ego* is reinforced, self-confidence boosts, and the girl starts to perceive herself as better, more original, perhaps even "superhuman." The anorexic who undertakes an almost heroic attempt to rise to a higher, almost divine, level of functioning is probably on the same path as the faithful striving for "spiritual development." So is it possible to speak of spirituality in anorexia?

Spirituality is beyond the individual's biological, psychological, and social systems. It is the possible transgression of the limits and restrictions of our human condition. Drastic refusal of food could probably mean transgressing these limits. However, the anorexic's goal is unrealistic. She cannot become an archetype. The anorexic approaches the described pattern only in an imagined way, through concentration on her *ego*. For a period of time, she may feel victorious when her artificial independence takes the appearance of true freedom. But it is so only until the somatic functions of the organism collapse. Then the girl may suddenly realize that she has not achieved anything, she has not defeated her body nor got rid of dependence on the world. This awareness, however, can save her from death. Origen in his *Homilies on Exodus* says:

> for no one is invisible, no one incorporeal, no one unchangeable, no one without beginning and without end, no one the creator of all except the Father with the Son and the Holy Spirit. (Quoted in Balthasar 2001, 56)

## NOTES

1. The term "archetype" was introduced to psychology by Jung. He states that archetypes "exist preconsciously, and presumably they form the structural dominants of the psyche in general. They may be compared to the invisible presence of the crystal lattice in a saturated solution. As *a priori* conditioning factors they represent a special, psychological instance of the biological 'pattern of behavior,' which gives all living organisms their specific qualities" (Jung 2014, 45). And in another work he writes: "They [archetypes] are, indeed, an instinctive trend, as marked as the impulse of birds to build nests, or ants to form organized colonies" (Jung 1964, 69).

2. As one can see, there is some structural similarity to obsessive-compulsive disorder here. Psychiatry also locates anorexia within the "obsessive-compulsive spectrum" of disorders.

3. According to Fromm, repression separates man, being a contingent person, a product of social conditions, from the being that can be referred to as the "universal man."

4. Compare with Feuerbach's considerations reconstructed in chapter 2.

5. There is a similarity to some elements of narcissism, schizoidism, and schizophrenia (see chapter 5).

6. The process is similar to the one described in the chapter that addresses obsessive-compulsive disorder ("mixing" of the part that *participates* with the outside).

7. Perhaps these phenomena contain elements that coincide with those of the primitive mentality that manifest themselves in *tjurunga*. A *tjurunga* ("secret," "sacred") is usually an oblong, ornamented piece of wood or stone which for a native Australian constitutes, in a sense, an extension of his own existence by his ancestors' "souls." Thus, the *tjurunga* is a part of a given person (see Szyjewski 2000, 175–84).

8. The family system of the girl suffering from anorexia often looks as follows. The mother is overburdened with bringing up the children and running the household,

she sometimes tries to combine both female and male functions and roles, but in fact she cannot deal with such a scope of responsibility. She often shows a specific ambitendency—on the one hand she manifests her reasonability and responsibility, and on the other hand she has the features of an immature, unfulfilled woman who refuses to get used to the idea that she is no longer a young girl. The daughter senses that her mother is weak, hurt, and frustrated. The father, if present in the family at all, has a rather poor contact with the daughter, which is often caused by his withdrawal from the relation due to his inability to adopt a proper approach towards her emerging genital sexuality (he fears his reactions to the daughter's sexuality, therefore he prefers to isolate from her). The parents lack a good relationship.

9. Being constantly focused on maintaining internal stability, anorexics often do not accept chaos and indeterminacy. Their day must be planned in detail. The day plan serves as protection against stimuli because a predictable day, defined and unsurprising, provides a stable framework that, in turn, makes it possible to fight the internal conflict. When the plan collapses, the sum of internal and external stimuli starts to exceed the organism's protection capabilities. The girl panics, foreseeing that she will not be able to deal with the threat of internal stimuli when they are combined with the external ones. The process is similar to the one occurring in obsessive-compulsive disorder, where the fixed external structure—in the form of compulsive rituals—protects from an external danger. For the same reason we put things around us into order which is to help us to reduce the chaos inside ourselves. Similarly, when we are exposed to, for example, a high level of noise, it is more difficult for us to control the internal agitation that results from an entirely different reason.

10. The *Self* is a category used by Jung to denote the archetype of wholeness, completeness of the psyche. It is, in a way, the center of the conscious and unconscious mind, the center of the entire person. The *Self* manifests itself in the form of archetypal images, such as the vision of God (see Samuels, Shorter, and Plaut 1986).

*Chapter Five*

# Psychosis, Narcissism, God

## SCHIZOPHRENIA—MESSIANISM, MANICHAEISM, AND SPHERICITY

### Schizophrenia—What Is That?

Psychosis is a state of detachment from social reality, it is confusion and inadequacy, a state of mental disorganization. It is also lack of self-reliance and real responsibility for others. However, psychosis such as schizophrenia may also be a state of increased sensitivity and often of specific insight.

Schizophrenia is not easy to describe. The problem occurs even when we intend to clearly distinguish the area of psychopathological phenomena defined by this term, and intensifies when we analyze its nature and genesis. If, desiring to capture what seems to be the most specific for this disease, we do not want to reduce it to a textbook presentation of group of symptoms, we must choose the elements of the picture, which means constructing some "schizophrenia."[1]

One needs to keep in mind that "schizophrenia" is not any particular being, but only the name we give to the group of phenomena that we want to identify as relatively unambiguous and repetitive. It does not exist as, for example, a stomach ulcer. One can say that the patient *has* an ulcer, but to say that the person *has* schizophrenia is much less adequate. Saying that someone *is* schizophrenic may also be confusing. "Schizophrenia" does not exist as physical objects, nor does it constitute the essence of any person.

If I recognize something from afar as a "chair," I know quite exactly what I will find when I walk up closer. I will gradually notice more and more new details: the shape of the backrest, the type of material, workmanship. However, it will always be, apart from impractical extravagances, an object to sit on, the shape and size of which are likely to fluctuate only within certain limits. So one can say that with the improvement of the perception quality, the chair acquires more details, but it still remains the chair. Now, with the formation such as schizophrenia it is otherwise. When I start to get to know it closer, it changes and can even cease to be "schizophrenia" in the generally recognized sense.[2] What schizophrenia is depends on our sensitivity in contact with the patient, the insight of observation, and the depth of refection. Officially, "schizophrenia" is a sum of observations and conclusions on certain events in the life of some people, that have been established and written in handbooks. However, the text does not describe the whole reality. Taking into account the most unequivocal cases, we have a fairly transparent and repeatable syndrome. However, in other cases, very specific structures heave into sight, which may require using a new name. Nevertheless, schizophrenia remains what the totality of physicians consider it to be. In other words, what an average physician can understand.

Eugen Bleuler, the author of the term, spoke of "a group of schizophrenias," and by such wording indicated the occurrence of differences in the picture of the disease. It should be noted that since the time the author lived, the criteria for diagnosing the disease have evolved (Wciórka 2002a, 219–25; Sadock and Sadock 2008, 156), which can basically be considered as the creation of new disease entities. Currently, to recognize it in a patient, one does no longer need to see Bleuler's axial symptoms, including two basic ones— autism and ambivalence. Present diagnostic manuals emphasize delusions, especially delusions of control or delusions of influence, and hallucinations (especially auditory), absentmindedness, or inadequate affect (see Sadock and Sadock 2008, 156). The differences in the diagnosis of schizophrenia also depend on a given country, e.g., narrow boundaries of schizophrenia are defined in France and the United Kingdom, and wide in the United States (Wciórka 2002a, 234; Moskowitz and Heim 2011, 471). Ultimately, the diagnosis depends on the subjective approach of a given psychiatrist (despite the seemingly clear diagnostic directions, there are frequent cases in which one physician will recognize schizophrenia and the other can give a different diagnosis). Generally speaking, schizophrenia has become a very capacious, probably too capacious, diagnostic category in which various psychotic states are placed (Wciórka 2002a, 225).[3]

## Schizophrenic Messianism

The picture of a man who imagines that he is a prophet, messiah, or God Himself has become a symbol of madness. Delusions of grandeur are very frequent in schizophrenia, although it is infrequent that a sick man has an extremely grandiose image of himself for a long time. This image rather fluctuates, and the patient is convinced of his unlimited power only sometimes. He may then believe he is "God" Himself or at least someone similar. Delusions of this type are this frequent because they play an important role within the dynamics of the disturbed mind. This function has two components: isolation and syntony that, though opposite, complement each other. The schizophrenic is isolated and tends to isolate, but this tendency also involves the compensating opposite one.

A delusion of grandeur, which usually takes the form of a delusion of mission, is a kind of compromise between isolation and being with people. Who else, other than a ruler, dictator, or messiah, is both different and alienated, and at the same time does not reach the margin of life, but—on the contrary—everyone feels his influence and connects with him in some way? The messiah is alone, but everyone sees him; he is in the center of the community. The stronger the isolation, the greater the mission must become for the people to be close after all. The greater the mission, the stronger the isolation may be. Both tendencies determine each other, because both have the same meaning for the psyche of the sick man. The greatness of the played character indicates the greatness of the isolation. If one can return to the world only as God and Savior, it means so much that the tendency to isolation has reached its zenith.

The mission provides a sense of meaning and identity, and the legitimacy of one's own existence. Being "God" gives a complete escape from the tiresome human relationships and conditions. The schizophrenic, becoming "God," frees himself from the embarrassing influence of the past, childhood, and family, gets rid of the family and the socially conditioned guilt, which is one of the factors constraining the freedom of the *ego*. Just as the cultural image of God is formed by eliminating the figures of parents, the schizophrenic, to break away from parents, becomes God.

Entering into normal relationships always involves some collapse of the sense of grandeur because it is only possible in case of accepting the value of others. The schizophrenic cannot live with people, neither can he—as a human being—live without them. To keep the valuable isolation, and at the same time, stay in touch with other people, he appears as someone surpassing them, but also having something precious for them.

Adam Wizel, a psychiatrist from Warsaw, published his patient's diary written during the First World War (Wizel 2001).[4] The author with an unknown name, a person isolated from people, and at the same time immersed in fantasies about her own mission (giving birth and upbringing of a genius), writes:

Oh earth, earth, I must leave my legacy to the future. I, I, I—I am the power. [. . .] People, here I am, unknown to you, indifferent, I vow to you today for the thousandth time that you will be proud of me. My enforced idleness, this tragedy of awaiting simply takes my consciousness away. The thought that I do not do anything great yet, that I can be at this moment at most "a good and honest person." But the future is mine, mine (Wizel 2001, 105).[5]

## Duality and Idealization

In schizophrenia, dividing people into "good" and "bad," "stupid" and "wise," "nice" and "ugly" is a frequently occurring scheme. This phenomenon, appearing clearly and regularly in the moments of the schizophrenic disorganization, proves that the idea of duality or polarity and the bivalent logic are deeply rooted in cognitive patterns. The schizophrenic feels the compulsion to make these Manichean divisions. Everyone must have their place at the poles of "good" and "evil." He divides people into "angels" or "holy" on one side, and "devils"—on the other (Kępiński 1992, 133). He also oscillates from pole to pole.

The process of emerging of the polarity, so characteristic in schizophrenia, can also be observed in some sense in transformations of certain religious ideas. Analyzing these ideas, we notice split and fusion of the "bad" and "good" poles in the image of the deity. There is no doubt that there are moments in the development of religion, in which the image of the deity is more "synthetic," it means it contains what is commonly called "evil" in our culture. The word *sacrum* itself means at the same time "holy" and "cursed." It is enough to look at the image of Yahweh, who is not only "jealous" but can be vindictive, ruthless, and uncontrollable. He is different from his later transformation, expressed in the Christian image of God—the Trinity. The concept of taboo (Polynesian *tapu*), commonly known in religious studies, means "holy" or "unclean" and "cursed" at the same time (Szyjewski 2001, 103 et seq.). It can express the *sacrum* as endowed with power (*mana*), and at the same time not indicate any ethical category.

Schizophrenic dividing resembles Manichaeism, in which there is a split into the "god of good" and "the god of evil," and the ontological equivalence of the two elements (Jonas 1994, 224–26). Some aspects of the schizophrenic process seem to show forces similar to those that can control the process of formation of Christian heresies. An element of the latter is the clarity of the division, introduced due to dissatisfaction with the Catholic dogmatics that keeps contradictions. Like the schizophrenic, these movements believe, that it is possible to reach the pole of the "good," the position of the "pure" (Cathars, the Puritans), the "perfect" (Albigenses), the angel-like (Angelics).[6]

The issue of the importance of duality for the human mind is complicated. It is puzzling, why the idea of the division of the reality into "good" and "evil" is so obvious, since every closer observation invariably suggests that nothing is arranged according to the divalent scheme. The theory of Melanie

Klein, and precisely what she called the paranoid-schizoid position (Segal 1974, 24 et seq.), may contribute to the search of sources of dual divisions in schizophrenia. The paranoid-schizoid position is the primary psychic structure consisting of defenses, anxieties and relationships with internal objects. It dominates in the life of a newborn, but remains deep in the psyche of every adult. Klein describes it based on the relation between the infant and the mother's breast. In this contact the child experiences pleasure and pain. The first, when being properly fed, and the latter when missing the breast. Unable to tolerate such different feelings, it splits the mother's breast into "two": the good and the bad. It idealizes the good, while the bad one becomes demonic (regardless of the details of the mechanism described by Klein, it seems logical that the child rather perceives "two" breasts than integrates opposing aspects of the breast in one object, as the second activity seems to require more mental operations). The same aspect of mental functioning is observed in schizophrenics. The schizophrenic cannot keep contradictions inside in the normal way, and to emotionally survive, begins a peculiar "eschatological" process, aiming at the final division of the reality into "good" and "evil" (Hinshelwood 1994, 98).

The phenomenon of bipolar splitting is associated with the idealization, in the sense of attributing an object extremely positive or negative values, for example as its "divinizing" or "demonization." It occurs constantly at the level of individual and social life.[7] Trying to comprehend the issue of stereotyping, let us refer to Claude Lévi-Strauss, who noted that perhaps the reduction factor is the primary reason for the aesthetic experience (Lévi-Strauss 1966, 22–25). For it seems that every reduction model has some aesthetic value. That is why we are pleased to see a miniature train, an aircraft model, or a few centimeters big, very similar to the original, chair. Lévi-Strauss suggests that probably in every work of art there is an element of reduction, although this does not need to be a reduction in size but a reduction of the properties. Painting reduces one of the spatial dimensions, sculpture—the color, the smell, the variety of tactile sensations. Both of these arts eliminate the time dimension of the object.

What does the reduction cause to the recipient that it becomes the core of the aesthetic experience? Lévi-Strauss states that we have here a kind of reversal of the process of cognition. Thanks to the reduction we are not bombarded with a great number of details, but we perceive the object at one time and in full. To quote the author's words:

> To understand a real object in its totality we always tend to work from its parts. The resistance it offers us is overcome by dividing it. Reduction in scale reverses this situation. Being smaller, the object as a whole seems less formidable. By being quantitatively diminished, it seems to us qualitatively simplified. More

exactly, this quantitative transposition extends and diversifies our power over a homologue of the thing, and by means of it the latter can be grasped, assessed and apprehended at a glance. A child's doll is no longer an enemy, a rival or even an interlocutor. In it and through it a person is made into a subject. In the case of miniatures, in contrast to what happens when we try to understand an object or living creature of real dimensions, knowledge of the whole precedes knowledge of the parts. And even if this is an illusion, the point of the procedure is to create or sustain the illusion, which gratifies the intelligence and gives rise to a sense of pleasure which can already be called aesthetic on these grounds alone. (Lévi–Strauss 1966, 23–24)

The same factors are responsible for the idealization of the images of people we have. The idealization enables simplification of the image and reduction of the immense amount of information to a simple scheme. We no longer have to associate with something varying in time, complex, constantly showing new details and evading unambiguous assessment. We grasp a picture with a single glance. This is exactly the reduced model, something similar to the sculpture, which, although portrays the external shape of a man, will not surprise us with a rumbling stomach or an unexpected gesture. The schizophrenic, creating the reduced world around, defends himself against the flood of unknown, impossible to comprehend stimuli (see Grzywa 2000, 108).

## Ambisentences and Sphericity

The image of schizophrenia indicates that we do not deal only with the disintegration of the unity of personality, but also with a parallel attempt of the psyche to restore the unity. Fighting for the consistency of personality, schizophrenia establishes very specific *coincidentia oppositorum*, namely the coexistence of opposites and contradictions. In schizophrenics' statements it is manifested through ambisentences characteristic of the disease, that is through expressing contradictory sentences at the same time. The patient says, for example: "My brother took care of me, he did not take care of me," or that he loves someone, and the next moment says he does not love this person. The second of the statements is not used as a negation of the first (by rethinking the issue, for instance), it is expressed *next to* the first. Many examples of ambisentences are found in the diaries of Vaslav Nijinsky, a great Russian (of Polish origin) ballet dancer, whose artistic career ended at the age of twenty-nine as a result of progressive schizophrenia. Here is one of them:

I like the fountain pen, as it is very handy. You can carry it in your pocket with the ink. It is a very cunning idea, since many want to have such a penholder. I do not like the fountain pen, because it is unhandy. I will write with it because I received it from my wife as a gift for Christmas (Nijinsky 2000, 62).[8]

The schizophrenic is afraid of declarations and choice, as this exposes to a conflict with the opposite statement. Expressing ambisentences, so characteristic of schizophrenia, is an attempt to establish the psychic unity. In this way, the schizophrenic tries to realize the archetypal image of God, that is—as Heraclitus said—"day [and] night, winter [and] summer, war [and] peace, satiety [and] hunger" (quoted in O'Connell 2006, 63). In such an image his psyche finds a moment of peace. We can say that through the coexistence of contradictions the schizophrenic tries to be "spherical," to not come into conflict and gain a sense of security.

I consider creating this kind of "sphericity" to be part of the *coiling-up* process. It is about this, what Jung called *circumambulation* (Samuels, Shorter, and Plaut 1986, 76), about the fundamental process for the psyche, the process of "encirclement" and the creation of the center. Jung found its expressions in the tradition of drawing a mandala, in the symbolism of the Christian Mass, in the work of a dream, and in the alchemical symbolism. In his view, this process allows the assimilation of opposites, preventing psychotic disintegration. The final "sphericity" is the *Self* that at the level of the archetypal image is identical to the theological vision of God. As one can see, even if the disintegration occurs, it does not cease to function—the schizophrenic's mental life reveals the effect of the *coiling-up* process even more clearly.

Theorems about God can often be illustrated with a model of sphere or circle. The medieval theologian Alan of Lille found the following phrase in the *Corpus Hermeticum*: "God is an intelligible sphere, whose center is everywhere and whose circumference is nowhere." And Nicholas of Cusa says, simply, that the whole theology "exists as circular and is based on circularity" (Nicholas of Cusa 1997, 95). Perfection of the circle and sphere hypnotizes.

Nicolaus Copernicus, in the first chapter of *On The Revolutions*, writes:

First of all, we must note that the universe is spherical. The reason is either that, of all forms, the sphere is the most perfect, needing no joint and being a complete whole, which can be neither increased nor diminished; or that it is the most capacious of figures, best suited to enclose and retain all things; or even that all the separate parts of the universe, I mean the sun, moon, planets and stars, are seen to be of this shape; or that wholes strive to be circumscribed by this boundary, as is apparent in drops of water and other fluid bodies when they seek to be self-contained. Hence no one will question the attribution of this form to the divine bodies. (Copernicus 1978, 8)

Aristotle concluded that the movements of the soul cannot be circular (see Stachowski 1992, 102), however, regarding the mind, he stated:

> We must identify the circle referred to with thought; for it is thought whose movement is thinking, and it is the circle whose movement is revolution, so that if thinking is a movement of revolution, the circle which has this characteristic movement must be thought. (Quoted in Stachowski 1992, 102)

Philo of Alexandria, referring to the "angels" moving stars, says that they move "in the manner most akin to intellect—the circle" (quoted in Wilson 2011, 186).

So not only God is spherical, but also the cosmos, soul, mind, reason. Do we deal with completely different things, for which the same metaphor was used accidentally? Or maybe it refers to the same reality? This reality would be a mental reality. The images of the sphere and circle are repeated, because they are based on a dynamic archetype. They are a projection of the universal "needs" and "strivings" of the psyche. Parmenides, searching for "the being," could find nothing but a sphere:

> It is completed on all sides, like the bulk of a well-rounded ball, equal in every way from the middle. (Quoted in Pellegrin 2000, 56)

When Empedocles describes *Sphairos*—the cosmos united in one by love—he also refers to the shape of a sphere: "he is equal everywhere, and boundless as a whole, Sphairos, rounded, rejoicing in circular stillness" (quoted in Furley 1987, 87). Let us note the psychological themes—*Sphairos* is lonely and joyful. Plato, speaking about the creation and structure of the universe in *Timaeus*—which he described as a living organism endowed with a soul—also mentions the shape of a sphere. Here is what he writes:

> And he [demiurge] gave it a figure that was fitting and akin to it. But for that animal that is to embrace within itself all animals, the fitting figure would be the one that has embraced all figures within itself, however many there are; so for this reason too, he worked it in circular fashion, sculpting it into the form of a sphere, the figure that keeps itself in all directions equidistant from its center to its extremities and which, of all figures, is the most perfect and most similar to itself, since he considered that *similar* is vastly more beautiful than *dissimilar.* (Plato 2016, 18)

Justifying the spherical form of the universe, he speaks, like Empedocles, of the "emotional" state of the world, actually presenting the narcissistic-schizoid pattern of functioning:

So he made it all smooth on the outside and gave it a rounded finish, and this for many reasons. For of eyes it had no need at all, since nothing to be seen was left over on the outside; nor of hearing, since there was nothing to be heard. [. . .] For nothing either went out from it nor went toward it from anywhere—since there *was* nothing—for the animal was artfully born so as to provide its own waste as food for itself and to suffer and do everything within itself and by itself, since he who put it together considered that the animal would be much better if it were self-sufficient than in need of other things. [. . .] And after he put soul at its center, he stretched her throughout the whole, even to the point of covering the body on the outside with her as with a veil; and so, as a circle turning in a circle, he established a heaven that was one, alone, solitary—able by itself, because of its excellence, to be company to itself and to stand in need of no one other at all, and sufficient unto itself as acquaintance and friend. For all these very reasons, he begat it a happy god. (Plato 2016, 18–19)

A theory, like the one of Plato, arises primarily as a result of mental speculation, and to a very small extent under the influence of observation. For this reason, it becomes a description of the mind rather than of the world. The theories described here, based on non-empirical premises, include similar images (sphere, circle). So one can state that what shapes them, is a universal "need"—something that demands to be expressed. What they build is not a vision of the world, but—which some of them clearly admit—the mind. The circle and the sphere are images of the intrapsychic *coiling-up* process.

Circle and sphere fascinate not only at the level of the rational mind, their picture is appealing and is also a real strength in the area of the unconscious. A person suffering from schizophrenia and—in a different way—people with other types of disorders try to achieve the status of a kind of "mental sphericity," ensuring maximum safety and a sense of control.[9] Such mental dynamics always involves some form of "narcissism," isolation from people and the world. In this context, we can also analyze such an unusual phenomenon as coprophagy in schizophrenic patients, i.e., eating their own excrement (Green and Kohon 2005, 52). By "connecting the mouth with the anus," the schizophrenic forms a circle, like the ouroboros, the serpent eating its own tail, the symbol of wholeness.

## NARCISSISM AND SCHIZOPHRENIA

### Narcissism

We will now analyze the structure of narcissism. Such an analysis has a value in itself, but it will also bring us closer to the understanding of schizophrenia. Although the current psychiatric classification separates psychotic disorders from personality disorders, which include narcissism, using the terms "schiz-oid" (*DSM-5*; *ICD-10*) or "schizotypal personality disorder" *(DSM-5)*, it admits that there are personality types that somehow correspond with what we observe in psychosis.[10] Below I present a hermeneutic continuum of dis-orders of the "schizoid" type. My point is to start with the experiences of a non-psychotic person and then move closer to the understanding of the expe-riences of a psychotic. The starting point here is "narcissism"—as presented below—because it reveals a significant number of phenomena remarkably similar to those observed in schizophrenia. A certain degree of narcissistic reactions cannot be unfamiliar to anyone. At the end of my theoretical con-tinuum, I do not place schizophrenia, but a theoretical construct which I have called schizoidism. It is formed of the common part of the above-mentioned schizophrenia-like disorders and schizophrenia.[11]

The concept of narcissism is ambiguous. The term is known to common language, determining the one that is "in love with himself" and is used in Freud's theory of libido. It was also used to refer to sexual behaviors (autoeroticism). Karl Abraham was the first to use the category of narcis-sism to describe the psychotic condition (see Laplanche and Pontalis 2006, 255). Using this concept, he described the basic psychological mechanism of dementia praecox (early dementia), consisting in the withdrawal of libido from external objects and directing it to oneself. Later, these concepts were adopted and developed by Freud, who described psychosis as "narcissistic neurosis" (Laplanche and Pontalis 2006, 258).

There are plenty of theories about narcissism as a personality disorder, or simply a particular psychic structure (see Symington 1993, 95 et seq.). Most of them emphasize the narcissist's emotional isolation and fantasies of om-nipotence, some the importance of the self-image. The diagnostic criteria for a narcissistic personality included in the *DSM-IV* did not describe the specific structure, providing an essentially trivial picture of an egoist.[12] The current description included in the *DSM-5* is closer to the position presented here, as it indicates that the narcissistic person strongly refers to other people who regulate his perception of himself and self-esteem.

According to the popular approach it is the "love of oneself," but this state-ment says little, and adopting it as the key of interpretation does not help to understand this disorder. We will start the reflections on narcissism by saying that narcissism is associated with: (a) increased self-monitoring, (b) the focus on creating a self-image (so if narcissism is "love," it is rather addressed to one's own image), (c) the desire for emotional self-sufficiency and autonomy. These elements are not independent, but more or less condition one another.

I regard point (a), that is, increased self-observation, as pathognomonic (and therefore basic) for narcissism, and I refer to such cases as narcissism in the strict sense. Other elements can be present in varying degrees. On the theoretical plane, we can bring these three elements to a common point, which is an attempt to negate what I call *the position of the other*. It is about the tendency to "eliminate" the existence of others. Of course, it is not about the physical extermination, or even fantasies about it, but about a kind of "suppression," involving an attempt to not see this basic fact that man lives as one of many. It is not about the negation of the physical other, but the other as a "place," or a center of autonomous opinions, desires and a point of view inaccessible to us.

## The Quasi-Observer

One of the basic characteristics of narcissism is a specific split of *self*, involving the emergence of psychic structure, which we can call the "quasi-external observer."[13] This entails important consequences for the functioning of the individual. He constantly watches himself, cannot stop thinking about himself and concentrate on the outside. The narcissistic person does not simply look at the other but tries to look at himself and the whole situation, "me—the other." He observes himself somewhat from outside, as if from the position of the third person.

Of course we all watch ourselves, and in relations we are aware of not only the external situations, but also ourselves. A narcissistic person has, however, an excessively strong desire to perceive his situation as a kind of an image seen from a distance. Such a person lives as if he were constantly watched by himself (also "eavesdropped" because he permanently perceives how his words sound). Perhaps narcissistic people happen to talk to themselves more often than other people (apart from cases of psychosis, dementia etc.). Narcissistic talking to oneself would be a kind of "distancing," like narcissistic "looking" at oneself, trying to take a certain, essentially impossible, position. A kind of being "outside of oneself."

The mechanism of striving to "see oneself through the eyes of the other" may take parapsychotic forms. A twenty-year-old, intelligent man during his psychotherapy experienced psychic phenomena, which were bordering hallucinations (I would call them unintentional visualizations with open eyes). He "saw" a figure standing a little behind on the left side of the chair he sat on. The figure had an identical look as him. He had never experienced this type of phenomena before, but he realized that he had always intensely watched himself when in the company of other people, and then two perspectives overlapped: his own and the figure's. This "person" joined especially when he was talking to people "unlike" him, as if speaking to the interlocutor (association at the request of the therapist): "You cannot give me anything, I do not want to give you anything, I do not want to talk to you" (a characteristic trait of narcissism, which is striving for identification, is revealed here—only this is valuable, which is similar to me).

Another patient, a seventeen-year-old boy, lying on a mattress in a body psychotherapy session, had a sensation as if he were watching the whole situation (himself and me) from above. Even when he closed his eyes, he was still "watching" the situation. It was difficult for him to clearly describe his experiences, but he presented this state as a kind of an overlap of two perspectives: an ordinary one and another related to the "observer" from above. A twenty-eight-year old woman experienced similar states, when she was playing with her peers as a child. "One of her parts was playing, the other was watching other children." Another young patient in a way "saw" her own face, perhaps even better than the face of the interlocutor, whenever she spoke to someone. Wizel's patient, already cited here, writes:

> Today, before the evening I felt really bad and I knelt to pray. At that moment I imagined that I was sitting on a chair and looking at myself kneeling. I just said "Lord, Lord," and it all seemed so false, such a screaming desecration, that I did not dare to pray any longer. I am now really suffering, but that "something," which hardly ever falls asleep in me, is watching me constantly, comments on each of my deeds and thoughts, and I am afraid to say: this "something" is actually me, and the rest of my being, my thoughts, the concepts are a book that I read with passion. I only pose to be a human, and I am no human. (Wizel 2001, 26)[14]

Narcissistic dissociation has a serious impact on the functioning in life. To illustrate this, let us use the following example, which reveals similar mechanisms, although it will not be considered as a sign of pathology: a person performing an activity suddenly distracts their attention from this action and says, "It's going well." What happens then? The person discontinues to be fully committed to the course of the activity, and instead begins to perceive "himself-and-the-performed-activity." He perceives himself as if from outside, from the place where assessment becomes possible. Usually in this case, the performance of the activity is disturbed or even temporarily interrupted.

In narcissistic people any action may be disturbed by permanent jumping from the activity itself to the reflection on the "oneself-and-the-activity" situation. The described process intensifies while in the company of others. The person then begins thinking hard, trying to somehow "see" what image of him the others have. He begins to control every move and attempts to modify the image by changing his actions. At the same time, due to such intensive self-observation, it seems to him that every movement transmits a great deal of information towards the environment. Unable to let this information escape in an uncontrolled manner, he increases control. This is how a vicious circle of disorganizing behavior begins.

## Creating an Image

The tendency to "see with the eyes of another person" is an attempt to negate *the position of the other*, that is the place in which no one is exactly who they are in their place. *The position of the other* is the area of the creation of independent images and opinions. Taking over what normally belongs to the other, the narcissistic person tries to eliminate this place to prevent the formation of a different point of view. The way to do that is striving to be the sole creator of one's own image. The narcissist tries to build so strong and suggestive image of himself that every other depiction of himself would have to give in and become just a copy of what he said about himself. He wishes that there was only one look and one image—his look and the image created by himself.

Narcissistic persons attempt to avoid incomplete and one-sided opinions on themselves, because they fear that partial information or superficial observations will create a "false," or simply an independent image of themselves. The following problem may occur: a person feels great tension due to the fact that someone will mistakenly recognize or classify him. One patient told me that he was very afraid to enter another school because someone could think he was its student. Similarly, when he entered another residential block, he felt the tension that someone could assume that he lived there. Of course, in both cases, it was not about any specifics (such as the prestige of the school, the quality of the building), but only about the incorrect recognition. Why is this incorrect recognition so important? Now, a person who mistakenly classifies the narcissist, remains with his knowledge, and the narcissist will not have any effect on it. A mental "copy" of the person will be created, a copy that does not suit what he knows about himself. The incorrect recognition is then an evident proof of the existence of *the position of the other* that narcissists want to annihilate.

Narcissists try to manipulate their image, to present it as a whole in every situation, and thus protect it against deformation from others. That is why these people are so often insistent in speaking about themselves, or on the contrary, isolate themselves, limiting the opportunity for the environment to form an opinion on them. There are two strategies for presenting oneself used by narcissistic people. The first is using highly generalized statements. The listener does not receive any "raw information" on the narcissistic person, and just the already developed judgments and assertions. The purpose is to prevent independent perception and evaluation. This strategy resembles the deductive reasoning—a small number of general "principles" has to be enough for the listener to form an opinion. The second strategy is similar to induction—the narcissistic person gives a lot of information that is supposed to create the desirable image in the mind of the listener. The aim of both strategies is to make everyone know only what the given person is willing to accept as true about himself.

Here we come to an important point, whose understanding is the way to understanding of many psychotic experiences. The narcissist is afraid that in the mind of another human being there is the cognitive representation of him, that is, a set of the ideas, opinions, and attitudes to which he has no access. That is why he interprets being recognized by someone, for example, as a kind of control over him.[15] He often reacts to the gaze in a particularly strange way. One can say that the narcissist feels that the gaze of another human takes something away from him, namely a part of knowledge about him. The narcissist fears that someone looking at him will perceive things that he does not see, and thus will have something unavailable to him.

One young man was terrified when a classmate said that she "figured him out." On the second day he behaved differently than before, as if he wanted to discourage her from further attempts to get to know him, showing that they lead astray. In the context of an understanding of psychotic disorders, it is important that the narcissistic person can feel almost torn by the representing images that exist in the minds of other people. Also this situation must be regarded as conditioned by a sense of threat from *the position of the other*.

## Feeling of Existence, Anxiety of Being

Narcissistic persons put a lot of energy in trying to create a stable identity. However, this is the facade identity, detached from their deeper essence. These people live with a sense of constant threat of loss of their self-esteem. This is because if their facade identity is disturbed, they will become helpless, at risk of inferiority. Their facade *self* is very dependent on the environment and situational context. Therefore, such people react to problems at work, for example, with such a deep depression, if the identity with the profession was the core of their facade *self*. One could say that a person without this type of disorder "loses his job," and the narcissistic person "loses a part of himself."

Narcissistic people can be extremely assertive in situations in which their facade *self* fits well in the context. However, in situations that have nothing to do with the facade *self*, they are often shy and lost. We would say that narcissistic people have a hidden "feeling of inferiority." But what exactly is behind this term, since these people can behave in a grandiose way? A more appropriate statement would be that narcissists have *a reduced feeling of existence*. While on the one hand they can regard themselves as gods, on the other hand they feel as if they were not even human. Wizel's patient writes:

> Now one can say that people are the masters, heirs of this land, that they are at home, and I am not at home, I came from somewhere. (Wizel 2001, 129)[16]

This, what others have spontaneous right to, narcissists have to work out and defend. Someone else can simply be, they still need to present themselves to continue being. Therefore, in situations where one can only *be*, and cannot present oneself, they feel so insecure. This is illustrated by the following example.

One young woman responded with great discomfort when someone was watching her behavior. She was constantly thinking that they expected a particular course of activities from her. The girl reported the following incident: when—during her hospitalization—a nurse turned to her with some request, she suddenly turned away and left. This behavior was completely illogical and done as if in amok. This trivial incident reveals the elements important for understanding of narcissism. Let us look at it closer. The nurse asked the patient to do something (to sit down and roll up a sleeve of her blouse, or anything else). In response, the girl quickly did something, but it was an inadequate action. What happened? To understand this event, one has to have in mind the narcissistic problem of the patient—the fear of being the object of observation. The normal course of the considered interaction would have been as follows: the nurse expresses the request, the patient listens to her, and once she understands what she is asked for, she does it. If she does not fully understand, she asks. In this case it was different, because the girl wanted to follow the recommendation as soon as possible and as correctly as possible so much that she started to act aimlessly. This is an important point, characteristic of narcissism.

This problem, which severely limits the social efficiency, stems from the anxiety of being observed. However, its essence is something we describe as "the anxiety of being." To not experience this anxiety, the narcissistic person wants to hide behind the action he performs. To achieve this, he earnestly desires to do it perfectly, because he hopes that in this way the action will become—let us call it so—nonindividual. Remarkably refined things seem to be determined more by objective factors than the creator's individuality.[17] That is why they will not say anything about himself.

Each narcissistic person in fact hides behind the facade of his image, which he often obsessively presents. He fears that somebody will perceive him through the activities he performs. In the described case, the anxiety that the facade will fall, that the patient will show herself to others, was so great that it completely disrupted the action. She tried to anticipate the nurse's expectations, wanted to do the task immediately, without hesitation or a moment of incomprehension. This would be the moment of revealing her *being*.

This *being* and anxiety related to it is difficult to describe, because perhaps only narcissism shows this aspect of man as a problem. It is a condition similar to the situation of being naked. When we are naked, we lose what we have tried to create through clothes; we can feel diminished and even "less human." These narcissistic—and, in a sense, weird—feelings lead us to understand other, deeper, psychotic feelings—of non-existence or depersonalization.

## Self-Determination

The last dimension of narcissism is the pursuit of isolation and independence from others, and the specific type of self-control. It is mostly about emotional independence—narcissistic persons desire that others are unable to affect their emotional state. One boy tried hard, so that nobody could influence his mood, he always presented himself as full of joy and optimism. He was brutally attacked once, but did not defend himself because he did not want to unmask anger (he exposed himself to beating with a baseball bat). If he had burst, he would have felt like a loser, because it would mean that someone managed to affect his internal state. But the boy was a stoic only seemingly—he let his repressed rage explode when he was sure he initiated it. Another person, a young woman, was terrified that her emotions could depend on other people—for example, by the fact that they upset her—that is why she tried to provoke, and then stop various emotions in order to have, in real situations, full control over them. It is important to realize that in these cases it was not about the estimable skill of self-control, but rather a pathological fear of spontaneity and dependence on others.

The emotional dependence, from which the narcissistic person escapes, should be understood in very real terms. It stems from the fact that the psyche has a participatory aspect, namely that a "part" of it in various ways is related to others. Looking at it from this point of view, it is not at all obvious that we can bear a relationship. Although we cannot exist without some form of relationship, every relationship means that we lose ourselves to some extent, that we become somehow "stretched" between ourselves and the other. A narcissistic person does not want to let this happen, unable to assimilate the existence of *the position of the other*.

To clarify this issue, let us use an example of adultery. The narcissistic person will deny betrayal, will isolate or avenge. However, he will not be able to listen to his partner, to take up the causes of the incident. Avoiding confrontation, he will try to prove to himself that the other person does not have a major impact on his emotional condition (understood broadly as his "mental existence"). Otherwise he would have to acknowledge that his emotions have an external pole, that they partly take place within the relationship. He would be forced to admit that he can deal with certain emotions only in a relationship, that he is related, and that he can achieve peace only by respecting the position of another human. However, this awareness enforces the acknowledgment of *the position of the other*, for which the narcissistic person is not ready.

Narcissistic persons feel such an extreme need for independence and self-determination, that the things average people do not even notice can become a problem for them. The already mentioned young boy had a strong aversion to mathematics, because it was an area he had no influence on, and because he had to subordinate to its results unconditionally. The fact that he had no influence on his coming into the world was also a problem for him, and for this reason he wanted to have control over the moment of his death, demonstrating suicidal tendencies. Another patient of the same age could not stand that "someone in a way wrote a scenario for him," that he feels sometimes "as if a man or woman wanted to control him." In this way, the fact that the root of his existence was his parents and not himself was intolerable for him. Wizel's patient noted during her illness in her diary:

Good God, have mercy on me, if I am to live, bring my health back without the help of people, without this insane humiliation. (Wizel 2001, 125)[18]

In the functioning of the narcissistic person, in attempts to annihilate *the position of the other*, we clearly see the desire to exist as an only being, fully independent from other beings. Such a person may not start to evidently express delusions of grandeur, but in his imagination he is never fully human, he is always a little "different." Adopting an attitude of negating *the position of the other* includes an element analogous with the primary attribute of the idea of God as a being that is sole and unrestrained by other selves and their demands. Therefore, no narcissist is far from the recognition of his divinity.

Narcissistic people have a permanent feeling of "self-distinctness." This feeling is sometimes tiring for them, but it can also become a source for experiencing their self-esteem and uniqueness. In relation to the world they adopt an attitude of a distanced observer, limiting contacts with people who seem distant and "unrealistic" to them. Narcissistic people sometimes say they feel as if they were separated from the world by armored glass ("As if I were from another universe," "I feel as if they were displayed on-screen at the cinema").

This perception of the surrounding reality can cause a specific sense of "incomplete reality" of the world, which entails sensations that can be described as solipsistic.[19] It is a compensating pole of the mentioned *reduced feeling of existence*. The narcissistic person oscillates between the feeling of his own "unreality" and the feeling that other people are "unrealistic." However, since there is no balance on the plane of contact, relationships with people are not experienced personally, but often as the category of "me—them." This entails stereotyping of others—treating people as identical—and, as a result, the deepening sense of one's own distinctness and alienation. This dynamics becomes the basis for creating of a proximal attitude, which in the long term may take the forms close to delusions. The narcissistic person feels as if he were marked, and may have the impression that even the people met recently see his "distinctness."

## SCHIZOIDISM AND NARCISSISM

We will consider schizoidism as parallel to narcissism, different from it mainly in intensity of symptoms. While in narcissism I emphasized the splitting off the *quasi-observer*, in this case, I will focus on the mechanism of splitting into the internal and external *self* (both mechanisms describe interrelated phenomena, we will treat them separately to keep the clarity). The schizoid person hides his internal (spontaneous, emotional) *self* behind a facade of the external *self* (Kępiński 1992, 204). The inner *self* is more residual, hidden, and unstructured, and the facade *self* is more chimeric and less integrated with the whole personality than in the narcissistic person.

We can imagine the described structure of personality as a form of a sphere, which includes another, smaller sphere. I will now present an example of therapeutic work, which showed this visual representation. The person referred to fell into a state of apathy at the age of twenty, ceased to be capable of long-term contact with people or arranging any matters. She felt that she could not talk spontaneously, she did not know what to say, could think of nothing. Any conversation made her extremely tired, because it required a tremendous effort to form sentences in advance, none of which was satisfactory. The experiences frightened her, because all contacts with people, even professional, seemed impossible. She did not suffer from clinical depression but narcissistic personality disorder close to schizoid disorder. Before the breakdown—as she defined it—"she was building her character," trying to be smiling, talkative, and outgoing. Since she was a child she experienced enormous stress when in contact with people, constantly observing herself and the reactions of others. Once she played her performance, she locked herself in her room and started studying or crying. Her parents had no idea about their daughter's feelings, as they got easily deluded by her false personality. So, in their opinion, she was a cheerful and outgoing person.

The outer personality formed a large sphere around the inner core. The big sphere was composed of smiles and conversations, contacts with people. This sphere was fragile and cracked, but being in its area allowed the awareness to escape from the inner sphere. For the inside sphere included, first and foremost, anger or even rage, aversion to contacts, and also boredom, apathy, and pain, that is why being in it was unbearable. Using the image of the sphere, we will also say that the outside one, though large, was of low density, and the one inside—of significant density. By this I mean energy content, the saturation of the life force of both areas.

The patient's current condition was a kind of her falling into the core *self.* In a sense, it was a state of contact with herself, but it was scary, because the real part was completely unbearable. It must be stressed: the inner *self* is not the "true" one in the sense of something healthy, which should just be released. The splitting into the external and internal parts causes that the first becomes fragile, without power, strange in a sense, and the second primitive and socially retarded, therefore unable to enter relationships.

The schizoid person, watching the outside of his personality in his relations with the environment, may experience a feeling of unreality or artificiality (e.g., the impression of being "lifeless" or "an android" (Kępiński 1992, 168–69). These are symptoms of depersonalization known to psychiatry. These processes certainly have many unclear elements, but every human being may share similar experiences. If a behavior is dictated by the environment, and an individual adopts it only superficially, they may isolate internally from this behavior, and not acknowledge it as their own. When they watch themselves during this behavior, they will feel that they are "artificial." One can have this type of impression in situations where the etiquette or convention requires particularly much from us (children forced by parents to say "Hello" experience the same once they "learn" to do it). The sensation, transient in the case of the healthy person, becomes very strong in the schizoid or schizophrenic person, as it refers to the majority of what he does and thinks.

Because of the described splitting and lack of spontaneity the schizoid individual has a sense of not having a stable identity. It is of course the same in narcissism, in which we see the *reduced feeling of existence*. To deal with it, narcissistic people do not just build their image, but also try to identify themselves with someone. If we assume that this is the beginning of the continuum, its end are psychotic symptoms, such as echolalia, echopraxia, or echomimia.[20] The equivalent of these phenomena in narcissistic persons is their tendency to copy gestures and minor behaviors of others (Symington 1996, 116-27). Identification is a way to deal with relationships. I consider this narcissistic *mimesis* as one of the attempts to annihilate *the position of the other*—the narcissist involuntarily tries to take over all the other's attributes, somehow generate the other in himself, and thus deny the other's autonomy.

On the other hand, these activities result from problems with the narcissist's own identity. The narcissist takes over others' gestures, because he has an impression as if they existed "more." In the case of the psychotics we will deal with the states of apparent resonance, or symbiosis with other people. I met psychotic people who had a feeling that someone understood them without words, that they formed one, so to speak. Similarly, the narcissistic person, with all his isolationism, can have the impression that he has met someone who is almost identical. There is nothing strange about it—he is able to stand the relationship only with the reflection of himself.

Narcissistic and schizoid persons often wonder how they should behave in a given situation, what would be "natural." They try to behave in accordance with their ideas about what behavior would others expect from them. They experience real fear of "disappointing" expectations, in the sense that they perceive destruction of someone's ideas about them as a disaster. These people can try to always be the same, when in a relationship with some person. They will then earnestly endeavor not to show the aspect of themselves that—in their opinion—does not fit in the idea of the partner. So if, for example, they meet someone at work, they will not show any of their family life, etc. What do we deal with here? With a great concentration on the images of us that others have. This phenomenon is significant, in principle, it is about the fear of the others' minds, the great embarrassment of the existence of "not-my" thoughts.

We observe a tense attitude towards the images and mental reality in both narcissism and schizophrenia. The difference is that the narcissist has a feeling that he can control his image and the content of the others' minds, while the schizophrenic feels overwhelmed by the images of others. This means that nothing but their minds bothers him. The psychotic person may feel that nothing can hide from the eyes and the influence of others. Psychiatry refers to this condition as delusions of control and delusions of mind being read. The narcissistic person protects himself from it when trying to negate *the position of the other*. Delusions of control are in fact the defeat in the struggle for the exclusiveness of his *position*—when *the position of the other* becomes of extreme significance. The man has the impression that others "know something" about him, "know" him, "have a plan" towards him. He begins to feel as if his existence "here and now" was weaker than the one that takes place in the minds of other people.

Since for schizoid persons even the thoughts and ideas of other people are the force that has a direct impact on their minds, everything coming from the others becomes a threat. These fundamental concerns are expressed in the resistance against being understood, loved, recognized, or close. The schizoid person isolates himself to keep the minimum sense of independence. We can clearly see that the isolation is a defense mechanism because in a sense the psychotic person is extremely open to others. Mental life is a state of oscillation between the poles of isolation and symbiosis; the sick person is different from the healthy one by the range of deviations on this scale.

The schizoid person does not have—as Ronald David Laing writes—ontological security (Laing 2001, 40 et seq.). This is expressed in his constant sense of threat regarding his own identity and subjective being in general. These feelings are similar to those experienced by a narcissistic person, and which I described as the *reduced feeling of existence*. The schizoid person, like the narcissistic one, feels that the foundation of his personality is something fluid and unstable. He is not enough "personified," that is why his *ego*, more strongly than in the average person, escapes from the body. The schizoid individual feels constantly "not at home," has the impression that the world belongs to other people, and that it was designed this way and not the other for their convenience. This is of course consistent with the feelings of the narcissist, who feels "different" and pushed into something that is not built for him.

Schizoid individuals, as often as narcissistic ones, have underdeveloped skills to undertake specific actions in the material world, which results from splitting of the inner *self* from the realm of the body and the area of the facade *self*. The schizoid person cannot really get involved in the actions in the world, because his "efferent" sphere (facade *self* + body) is not related to the inner *self*, which could provide a real volition and affective commitment. The sense of disembodying observed in schizophrenia (e.g., walking above the ground, lack of body sensation) indicates the impairment of practical-life side of the functioning. Awkwardness may, as in narcissism, increase in the presence of other people. Sometimes the blockade is so great that the person has a feeling of emptiness in the head, does not know what to do completely.

The etiology of this type of mental dynamics is similar in narcissism. One girl was afraid to say anything to someone in the presence of her mother. Every word, gesture, or story of that girl made her mother utter opinions, which she was never able to correct. In the presence of others the mother always spoke on behalf of her, she always knew what her daughter really wanted, etc. The mother's attitude had lasted since the daughter's early childhood—which can be defined as an attempt to avoid confrontation with the distinctness and autonomy of the child—can cause that the child will have the impression of being "scanned," controlled, totally dependent on the mother. At the same time it will feel that the mother's eyes, although so penetrating, do not touch its real inner *self*. This area, not accepted by the parent, will also be repressed and rejected by the child.

**Table 5.1.   Relations of narcissistic and schizoid structures and symptoms**

| Narcissism | Schizoidism |
|---|---|
| splitting of *self*—facade *self* | splitting of *self*—facade *self* |
| *quasi-observer*—parapsychotic phenomena ("seeing oneself"), talking to oneself | *quasi-observer*—autoscopic hallucinations, commenting voices |
| unstructured areas of personality—fear of being watched, frequent feeling of confusion | unstructured areas of the personality—difficulties and awkwardness in social situations |
| lack of spontaneity, feeling of embarrassment, "not being oneself" | depersonalization (feeling of being an android, dead, etc.) |
| disorganization of intentional actions | extreme disorganization of intentional actions |
| concentration on the mental representation of oneself created by others—sensitivity to others' opinions and ideas about oneself | "fear of others' minds"—delusions of mind being read and delusions of control |
| *the reduced feeling of existence*, feelings of emptiness, identity crisis compensated by grandiose fantasies | fear of annihilation (no ontological security), delusions of non-existence as well as of grandeur and mission |
| solipsistic feelings, isolation, lack of deeper relationships | autism, derealization |
| a sense of being "different" and ideas of references, the attitude "me—them" | delusions of reference and persecution |
| narcissistic *mimesis* | echolalia, echopraxia, echomimia |
| tendency to stereotypically judge people | obsessive dual divisions |
| etiological factor: lack of acceptance (threat) and / or perception of the spontaneity-individual sphere of personality | etiological factor: threat for biological existence of the individual, lack of acceptance and / or perception of the spontaneity-individual sphere of personality |

*Source:* Damian Janus.

Table 5.1 presents the relations of the narcissistic and schizoid structures and symptoms. It should be taken into account that many of the elements shown therein, determine one another and intertwine.

## THE TRUTH OF DELUSIONS

### Delusion: An Ambiguous Phenomenon

The psychiatrist treating psychosis in the context of pharmacotherapy usually is not much interested in the content of delusions. He should not, however, disregard the form in which the patient presents himself, because it can be very diverse and tell a lot about the depth of his pathology. Generally it must be said that patients are immersed in their delusions to varying degrees, even if their content is similar interindividually. It means that particular persons can experience them stronger or weaker, and be more or less distant from their content. The degree of experiencing delusions creates a continuum. At its one end there is a person who expresses his imaginary opinions with full assertion and conviction, at the other—someone who says: "I have the impression as if these cars drove up here on purpose, as if there were some people who are supposed to go somewhere, pass some information about me or something like that" (let us note that this person does not say: "They came to spy on me, they provide information about me to the KGB"). In the course of psychotherapy delusions can be dissolved and manifest only in the latter form. In turn, the psychiatrist, who (during the anamnesis) concentrates on finding particular elements necessary to issue a diagnosis can make the patient express them with more confidence.

Many types of delusions reoccur in very similar forms, which leaves no doubt that the forces conditioning them must be culturally universal or are existentially important. Psychiatric observation shows that the diversity of the content of delusions is not unlimited, and the vast majority includes just a few topics. These basic topics are: jealousy, guilt, belief of having power or mission, delusions concerning the functioning of the body (fantastic diseases, lack of function or non-existence of internal organs, etc.), the feeling of being watched, controlled or persecuted, delusions concerning various forms of access to psychic experiences in the form of reading, taking away or insertion of thoughts by others (Grzywa 2000, 236).

Closer observation indicates that many delusions are often formed based on strong feelings. It may then be so that someone does not "imagine" that the mother affects them telepathically, but they clearly feel it. The question, to what degree it is "purely subjective" and to what degree physical factors play a role here, is open (see Eisenbud 1970).

## Delusion as a Transformed Need

Freud's known schema shows persecutory delusions as arising from the homosexual needs and anxiety of them (Freud 1997d, 153 et seq.). This schema is as follows: "I desire him" becomes the defensive "I hate him," which in turn is projected and takes the form of "he hates me." I think that the schema, not being incorrect, is too narrow. More broadly, the delusion of persecution arises as a result of the general need for contact with humans. For a persecuted person should not complain about the lack of interest in them.

In order to investigate the basic mechanism of delusions, let us imagine a living alone, aged person.[21] It happens that such people claim that thieves secretly steal sugar from them, or that neighbors lurk for their clothes lying useless in the drawers. Sometimes these people are not physically alone, but because of intellectual weakness and falling out of the rhythm of life are mentally and emotionally lonely. However, life in the void is not possible. *Horror vacui* becomes the driving force behind building one's own, imaginary world. But here there is a problem: this world cannot become populated with the philanthropists and guardians, because it would be too unrealistic. The psyche follows here, after all, the principle of economy and realism, and therefore chooses the most likely situation—ill-intentioned people. Their figures can also contain the projected aggression towards the rejecting, cold world.

We can analyze another model of formation of delusions based on the example of an imaginary adultery (Freud 1997d, 152–53). A person overwhelmed by such delusions, usually a man, groundlessly accuses his partner of infidelity. He watches her constantly, mistrusts her, makes excuses, and tries to catch her in the act. Observing the functioning of such a person, we have the impression that he wants to catch the partner cheating more than to find out that the accusations turn out to be wrong. So apart from the pain of jealousy there is a desire to discover the woman's sexual relationship with another partner. Jealousy is not possible to dissuade, because it is fed by this unrecognized and unappeasable desire. The desire brings another man in the relationship. Where does it come from?[22] The man wants to see the "real" sexuality, recognizing his own as infantile. Therefore, no one will dissuade him from the belief that the partner prefers someone else. The true sexuality takes place in the relationship of his partner with the imaginary lover—someone more attractive, more capable sexually, wealthier. Sometimes it is the partner's father or the patient's father (Kępiński 1992, 113). This man is torn: he suffers from the partner's alleged infidelity because he desires the infidelity strongly. He curses for infidelity, but he will not accept the idea of loyalty. What it is worth noting is the existence of the desire under the layer of fear.

## The Synchronic and Diachronic Aspect of Delusions

The meaning of imaginary content can be read on two levels, which we will call diachronic and synchronic. The diachronic side of a delusion involves its processed meaning, that is, the psychodynamic-symbolic meaning. The synchronic side of delusional assertions lies in their direct adequacy. Let us consider it based on an example of a patient with the delusional syndrome. This man had typical, complex delusions of persecution that persisted for many years. He complained about the neighbors, cursed them, claimed that they robbed him, poisoned him with gas, and let insects in his apartment. In his stories, he often mentioned the situation in his previous workplace—he felt harmed by others who had various pacts with one another and settled affairs behind his back. He constantly felt that the others plotted against him. We can say that other people were somehow related to one another in his eyes, that they formed a kind of community, helped one another, ignoring him or harming him at the same time. What is the origin of this feeling?

The patient in his infancy lost both parents, who were killed by the Nazis during the war. Later, his grandmother raised him, and after her early death he was sent to an orphanage. His delusions were an expression of loneliness and lack of a sense of belonging. Because he was lonely and acutely felt his loneliness, he created people who were constantly interested in him. In addition, he felt that others stuck together, looked after one another. These feelings came from the fact that he was never a family member and did not experience its support. Those others who helped themselves at his expense, were like members of the same "family" he did not belong to, because he never belonged to any family. These are diachronic aspects, relating to the patient's past and expressing his internal structure in a processed way.

Let us now focus on the synchronic aspect. It is expressed in the fact that, from a certain point of view, this man had the right to say that the neighbors were hostile to him. They said in defense that "they have nothing against him," "they do not get in his way," "they are not interested in him." Their hostile attitude was expressed in indifference, which they did not want to admit, insisting on the assertion that it has no negative aspect. In reality, however, indifference is always close to hostility, which this man felt so strongly. We can explain this aspect of delusions, providing another example.

One patient defined his psychiatrist as "Antichrist," he said: "These are not my delusions, he wants to control me or kill me." The doctor, of course, treated his patient's claims as absurd, and he communicated it to him. However, the patient insisted on his statements, constantly repeating them. It was enough, however, to try to understand him and say: "I see that you feel incapacitated, depending on the doctor. That there is a conflict between you," and the patient uttered the words, "Yes, maybe he is not the Antichrist, but he is a very bad man." In fact, the doctor had a lot of repressed aggression towards the patient who, by his attitude, questioned his masculine-medical power. Of course he did not express these emotions directly, but in a passive-aggressive way, by avoiding full contact with the patient, the lack of serious attitude towards his words, and rigid adherence to his original recommendations. So the sick person used "demonology" to express what actually happened, although under the cover of factual and favorable therapeutic contact.

## Decoding and Discovering Delusions

In the approach to delusions we can distinguish an aspect of their decoding and—let us call it so—discovering. Decoding consists in treating the patient's language as a code, which should be translated into intelligible speech. The case of the "Antichrist" above is an example of this procedure. Another example may be the experiences of a patient who was prescribed electroshock. The woman's behavior indicated that this method of treatment alone did not solve her psychological problems. However, the doctors developed an attitude of "objective necessity," seeing it as the only treatment intervention they had in this case. The patient was alone with her "subjective" needs and fears, without the possibility of communicating them to anyone. During this time, she began to have delusions that they wanted to strangle her in the hospital. Despite persuasion, she persisted in this idea. It is not difficult to see that she expressed the interpersonal reality—the staff "strangled" her by refusing to take her feelings and fears seriously (later on she also imagined that "she would end up in an electric chair"). Assuming an objectified understanding of a mental illness—expressed by the belief that an electric shock may improve brain functioning—the doctors did not want to notice that they led the psyche into the state of extreme anxiety and confusion—the same psyche that was intended to be healed by treating the brain.

Discovering delusions is something more complex, involving the constructivist nature of knowledge.[23] In this case, the patient's language cannot be clearly translated into the universal language. The patient talks about things for which common means of communication are insufficient.

Let us take an example of anorexia. Probably everyone who had anything to do with a person suffering from anorexia has heard her irrational statements concerning "being fat." A fully intellectually functional person, pointing at her emaciated body, states that she is "fat," sometimes also claiming that she is "fatter" than others from her environment.[24] The arguments that she is not "fat" are pointless; they do not eliminate the fear of gaining weight and aversion to her "fat." In many cases, this type of anorexics' claim can be qualified as close to delusion. They are objectively false opinions that cannot be modified by rational argumentation. However, if our reasoning is not accepted by the anorexic, if it varies from what she says and experiences, it makes us suppose that each party is talking about something else. The anorexic does not speak of the same "being fat" that the healthy person means. Her words cover another area of experiencing, not fully available to the person without anorexia. What is this area? The anorexic, saying that she is "too fat," says something near the statements: "I am not enough skinny," "I can be evaluated," "I cannot accept my body, which is not in the process of weight loss," "I am frightened of the possibility of sudden, almost magical weight gain," etc. Of course what the anorexic really experiences is still "next to" these terms, but they are certainly closer to her situation than the conventional notion of "being too fat."

To adequately describe the mental life, we need to create new understanding and new concepts. Words and styles of understanding that we use every day are not always enough. To describe man, it is not enough to use terms like "he thinks that," "he loves," "he hates" and so on may be insufficient. Also, a more complicated approach, using statements like "he is afraid of his own aggression," "he unconsciously identifies with his mother" etc., has only a limited degree of adequacy.

Let us consider the following statement: "He is experiencing depression because of separation from his wife." Perhaps this sentence seems to be quite precise and logical, giving an understandable reason for a certain mental state. And it would often be the end of our investigation of the case. It could also be the core of the identity of the ex-husband as a "poor, abandoned man." However, the "cause," which this sentence presupposes, is not necessarily—and to some extent, is certainly not—the cause of the mental state of the man. A "sorrow-for-his-leaving-wife" is a picture, a compact construct subjected to stereotyping, which functions within the area of social communication. Hearing about it, we know immediately what it is about: People love and need each other, when one leaves, the other experiences a sense of tremendous loss, and so on. In fact, what functions as a "sorrow-for-his-leaving-wife" always hides dozens of subtle and implicit elements. If I name them, of course, I will not definitely enlighten the "real reasons," and I will only avoid extreme simplifications. Here are the possible components: the narcissistic trauma, the revived memory of losing Mother, a sense of lost time and meaninglessness of the world, suppressed rage, a sense of losing a part of oneself, and so on. Another illustration of what is mentioned above is the functioning of the phrase "I love you." When we watch a film with a love theme and we eventually hear "I love you," we have the impression that now it is all clear, that what had been happening between the two characters finally gained a certain clarification. These words create such a strong complex of meanings in our culture that after hearing them we kind of cease to observe the true reality. But every "I love you" is different, depends on who says it, and in what situation. Therefore, we actually still do not know what is happening between these two persons. It is similar with the definition of "love."

I mentioned the examples concerning human relationships, because in these cases, our tendency to "hypnotize ourselves" with words is particularly strong. One can say that we not only think *with words*, but somehow we think *about them*. Instead of using them only as tools enabling our contact with reality, we stop at them. "Stratification" of language and reality exists. Ludwig Wittgenstein noticed it. Here is what he stated:

> Suppose that the question is "what do you mean by that gesture?" and the answer is "I mean you must leave." The answer would not have been more correctly phrased: "I mean what I mean by the sentence 'you must leave'. [. . .] But if you say: "How am I to know what he means, when I see nothing but the signs he gives?" then I say: "How is *he* to know what he means, when he has nothing but the signs either?" (Wittgenstein 1978, 40)

It turns out that talking does not present reality, in this case—psychological processes. The psychological interpretation—of this extremely simple behavior—saying that the man *means* that someone should leave, is correct only in a limited extent. Both speaking and gestures are immersed in a broader process of life, which is not fully verbalized and possible to communicate verbally.

Let us approach these issues from yet another side. The process of discovering delusions is parallel to the process of assimilation of ancient philosophical and scientific statements. If in antiquity one stated that everything consisted of four elements—water, fire, earth, and air—the modern physical chemistry has not revised these statements. Simply because the "water" then was another water than our $H_2O$, just as the "fire," "earth" and "air" of that time are not the same we know today. And it is not just about the differences in naming the same, constant elements of reality, but about a much less trivial process. Fleck, considering the eighteenth-century statements saying that a man with an empty stomach is heavier than after a meal, writes:

> Our physical reality did not exist for them. On the other hand, they were prepared to regard many another feature as real which no longer has meaning for us. (Fleck 1979, 127)

However, the difference between the old thought style and the modern one does not mean—as Fleck points out—that we know better and they were wrong, because the former authors had more to say and had better knowledge about what was more valuable to them.

So one can say that we now live in a reality different from the one in which our ancestors lived, and therefore we are not able to fully verify their statements. The belief that we have access to the entire natural experience of the past times, plus the contemporary experience is an illusion. In other words, the progress of knowledge in a broad sense is not strictly cumulative—some real knowledge becomes forgotten because of changes of the cultural sensitivity. That is why, for example, our contemporary assessment of astrology, magical and herbal medicine, or occult philosophy may not be exhaustive. We will simply not notice their former practical and explanatory features, at best these, which we will relate to the current experience (e.g., popular explanation of the magic with suggestion). What I say does not mean a complete relativism in assessing the level of knowledge of the world in various eras. In my opinion, the situation amounts to the fact that the total pool of information is now incomparably greater than that which existed in the past, it happened, however, at the expense of abandoning certain paths that people once tried to explore.

One cannot speak of the "constant elements of reality" because they are always the "perceived elements of reality" and what is perceived, is changeable, is a function of the evolution of science, culture and society. Fleck gives an example of the old (dated 1815) claims concerning the role of "phosphorus" in the body (Fleck 1979, 128–29). A physiologist of that time writes about phosphorus as a component of urine, but describes it as "a ferment of death," "the basis for food" or "the most perfect product of the animal life process." However, translating these statements into the current knowledge of the biochemical function of phosphorus in the body will not give us a proper image of the former science. And it is because our present "phosphorus" is different from "phosphorus" that author wrote about (on the other hand, the "contemporary" phosphorus has some properties of the old "phosphorus," such as that it is a component of urine). The ranges of both concepts (the old and the contemporary definition of phosphorus) are analogical but are not identical. The contemporary science has determined a certain area of experience, which it named "phosphorus," it found that this is an element and identified its various functions in the body. But certainly it lost other potential ways of recognition of experiencing "phosphorus," which its old concept showed.

Just as with delusions—translating them into generally comprehensible language enables communication, showing the meaning of the expression, but it also leads to the loss of subjective experience, for which there is no place in the universal linguistic convention. It simply does not exist in our socially constructed reality. This does not mean, however, that it is mere nothing.

## The Schizophrenic's World—Interregnum Between Paradigms

All knowledge has been constructed, and therefore nothing compels us to this, and no other presentation of reality. When I sit in an armchair, in a room familiar to me, to see something new, I do not have to wait for new stimuli to reach me from the outside. If, somehow, my cognitive categories change or widen, I could be flooded with a whole new vision of reality in an instant.

This indeed takes place sometimes. For example, when looking beyond the horizon marked by the vision of retirement, or beyond the vision of "heaven" composed of the unreflective certainty, we suddenly realize the fact of our transience deeper and sharper.

This, in another form of course, also happens in science during changes in prevailing paradigms, and in art, when the optics of presenting the world alters. In painting, a new direction is generally not associated with finding a new object of the pictures, but often with finding a different way of seeing, which reveals hitherto unnoticed dimensions.

The same happens in schizophrenia. What the schizophrenic experiences, and how he behaves, is the result of the partial deconstruction of the conventional or paradigmatic area of perception and communication. In paranoid schizophrenia the man is flooded by poorly structured information, which happens in the moment of separation from the socially fixed categories, meanings and definitions (Kępiński 1992, 163). As a result of this separation a kind of "paradigm change" happens, that is opening up to the possibility of a new view of the reality, and thus noticing new facts. The schizophrenic in this respect is similar to a researcher who has to put the old theory aside, because he cannot express the meaning of the new observations within it. This is where neologisms, so frequent in schizophrenia, come from—they are supposed to express what was inaccessible to knowledge before. Schizophrenics' "absurd" statements have their origin in the constructivist nature of knowledge (and in the fact of the opacity of human relationships—which is discussed below). Constructivism means that what we know about ourselves and about others can always be reformulated.

The schizophrenic is not all wrong; listening to his speech, we can find reality. Statements of people in schizophrenia may directly express content that for a normal person exists only on an unconscious level. They can, for instance, relate to the Oedipal conflict. Such a patient may explicitly deliberate the willingness for a sexual relationship with his mother and the hatred for his father.

The Oedipus complex is one of these elements, which we may not directly recognize in our lives, but which were already discovered by psychoanalysis.[25] Many other, seemingly incoherent, statements of schizophrenics are the expression of perceiving new, yet unexplored and not assimilated socially and linguistically elements of human reality (Wróbel 1984, 245; Grzywa 2000, 149).

Jacques Lacan said that the psychotic is a subject "who is *not duped by the symbolic order*" (Žižek 1992, 79). The real psychotic touches the Real that escapes symbolization and does not belong to the world of symbolic interactions, although it has a crucial influence on them. The eruption of the

Real is for example a sexual intercourse, an act that can never be expressed adequately—it is always idealized and romanticized or vulgarized, simplified and trivialized (let us analyze, for instance, how little the words "love" and "a lover" tell us about the real "activity"). Lacan's observations regarding the psychotic subject—despite all the differences, which I will not be dealing with here—show the same aspect of psychosis, which I am trying to describe: the psychotic is out of the convention, the words and their meanings do not have this "binding force" for him, as it is in the case of the neurotic and other people.

Due to the amount of information, the insufficient ability to process it, and because of withdrawal of the area of intersubjective communicability, the schizophrenic does not become an explorer or a true philosopher. He can never clearly express his cognition to us. The schizophrenic is certainly wrong in many points in his vision of the world, but we are on the other pole of the error. The common perception of reality, provided by the social habit, supported by defense mechanisms, causes that we tend to excessively make the world "normal." We do not see the murmuring background of our existence, the "*il y a*," that Emmanuel Lévinas wrote about (Lévinas 1991, 31–34), we are not aware of hidden messages circulating among people, we suppress fundamental questions. It is obvious to us that the schizophrenic vision is a "distortion of reality," as if we had some reality in our hands.

To understand schizophrenia, we must realize that the absurdity of schizophrenic statements is not an absolute absurdity. These statements are *completely* absurd *for us*, in the context of the current linguistic convention. However, assuming a certain point of view, we cannot say that the schizophrenic breaks the objective obviousness, and that the normal person does not. When in fact we look closer at our statements, it turns out that they are not so different from his "delusions."

Take, for example, a scientific theory which says that schizophrenia is caused due to disturbances in synaptic transmission.[26] In the sense I wish to present here, its acceptance would be similar to a delusion. This theory contains pertinent observations concerning some chemical changes in the brain accompanying schizophrenia and the ability to influence its course chemically. But this is not the same as the "basis" or "cause." Each "basis" and each "cause" is relative, it is a basis and a cause only in the scientific context. And thinking in terms of "causes"—one might say "absolute causes"—which appears here, upgrades relative components of the biomedical knowledge to the level of metaphysical assertions. After all, saying that about "causes" of mental disorders, we also speak about the nature of the psyche and the nature of man, reducing it to the current biochemical knowledge!

Also in past centuries people spoke on similar topics from similar perspectives. Currently, those statements seem to us funny, and some call them "delusions."[27] Most of those former assertions had a grain of truth, just as the present ones do. However, due to changes in our way of perception and thinking (change of paradigm, culture, language, way of life, etc.) what we see first is the layer of errors and inadequacy. The same can happen when someone reads our theories of the biochemical etiology of schizophrenia in three hundred years. They may not pay much attention to the reasonableness of some modest results, but focus on the inadequate extrapolations and simplifications. And eventually they may regard it all as incorrect.

## Non-Transparency of Relations and Delusions

The schizophrenic is someone particularly "sensitive" to what in human relations is hidden and pushed into the background. He is sensitive to all the unconscious messages coming from inside the family. These unconscious interactions between the family members, even if they are not one of the causes of psychosis, certainly modulate its course and form the symptoms. The schizophrenic is so much sensitive because he is "trained" from his earliest years to not trust the superficiality and look under the veil of appearances.

One can recall Gregory Bateson's theory of the double bind (Bateson et al. 1956). It says that a child who later on develops schizophrenia simultaneously receives two contradictory messages from its mother. One of them is overt, the other is always concealed. The first message may be verbal and the other arising from the mother's body language. She can, for example, say "I love you" only when she turns away from the child physically, increases bodily distance, etc. The mother behaving like this is "split," she is inconsistent in her actions towards the child. The child as a result learns that a man is not a solid whole, and being exposed to the mother's coldness, which is not confirmed by her words, discovers that hidden things may be more important than what is explicitly declared. The mother says that she loves, and maybe even believes in it and tries to make it so. Yes, she often actually loves the child. But the expression of her love can be so crippled by her own unconscious problems that what reaches the child will never be satisfactory for it. The mother becomes split for the child, as if now there were two "mothers." Which "mother" is the child supposed to trust now?

But it would be wrong to say that the family situation in which the schizophrenic lives is indeed qualitatively different from that of any other man. What we have said about the schizophrenic's family situation merely indicates and highlights the elements inherent in every interpersonal relationship. Man is not able to fully control everything that he brings into relationships with others, nor is he ever quite aware of the nature of things that have an effect on him in a given relationship. Regardless of the etiology of schizophrenia we must realize that *opacity* is a constitutive element of all meetings and interpersonal communication, and as such is a factor in forming the image of this disorder.

In one patient the first, as we can now reconstruct it, manifestations of schizophrenia were his niggling questions, which he addressed to his mother: "How do you recognize who is your friend and who is an enemy?" It may seem to healthy people that the answer is not that difficult or that the question is not even worth asking at all. They will find the schizophrenic's uncertainty about so obvious things strange. But the schizophrenic's doubts are not groundless. They begin at the moment when the person realizes that human relationships are—to put it mildly—very confusing, that, for example, the name "friend" is nothing clear, and does not protect from the fundamental indefiniteness.

What does the schizophrenic perceive exactly? He sees (or perhaps it is better to say that he "receives" because this kind of reception does not need to be associated with realizing) that the side that people directly and openly show each other is not their only one. He also realizes that human relationships are not based solely on what people participating in them declare. The schizophrenic sees masks around and is afraid of what lies beneath them. He can neither accept the social game nor cope with what he vaguely sees beneath it. He does not want masks, he feels lonely among them, and at the same time he is scared the masks could fall.

I would like to emphasize that these are not only distant metaphors. The world of relations really is a world of masks and games. A mask is a medium in each relationship. Normal people know how to live with it, the schizophrenic does not. Take an example from everyday life. A salesman is elegantly dressed, praises the goods, talks about the benefits of the purchase, smiles, is extremely polite. Let us notice the pose of his body: the legs together, stiff and straight in the knees, he leans forward slightly. If he does not hold the goods in his hands, he joins them. His pose is an example of an expressive mask. It is to convince the client about his unselfish intentions. The presented kindness, goodwill, and body posture confirm it. He joins the legs and tilts the pelvis backward to hide the aggression and instinctive greed (the legs apart and the pelvis pushed out would be an evidence of aggressiveness, desire for domination, and a selfish search for sexual satisfaction). Although we are aware of the fact that this man is "not fully himself," we can converse with him, and sometimes even enjoy this contact. In this we differ from the schizophrenic—he would not stand such a relationship. "The salesman" is a hyperbole, which shows a common fact—none of us and never is fully ourselves, everyone hides themselves, however much they swear they are sincere. I would say that a human "in himself" does not exist or is by all means unclear. This fundamental indeterminacy scares the schizophrenic, it is the essence of his interpersonal anxiety.

In relations, there always happens more than one can see, and what one consciously perceives is a function of the social, historical, and biographical context.[28] To some extent, what we say about ourselves, others, and our relationships has a defensive function. It defends us on the one hand from the indefiniteness and ambiguity of our existence, and on the other from its dark side, which we cannot even show to ourselves. Psychoanalysis or a deeper self-reflection reveal the deposits of terrible and antisocial things that each man carries inside him. The social convention protects us from realizing these matters.

The schizophrenic is afraid of the evil manifesting itself in both a positive and negative form, that is, respectively, aggression and loneliness. Any contact with another man exposes him to confrontation with these, hidden behind the mask, components of human existence (aggression or indifference). On the other hand, the schizophrenic cannot function at the level of social convention that, besides defense mechanisms, is the protection of average people (Kępiński 1992, 168). For him, our carelessness is truly crazy, yet each of us is exposed to potential aggression from all the others.[29] Not only "mortal enemies" are agressive with each other, it is possible and inevitable in every relationship. Even the relation of mother to child will never be free from it. We had the opportunity to see the strength and commonness of human aggression also not through analysis and introspection, but quite visually, embodied in the Nazi genocide.

Another problem is the problem of loneliness. Each person strives to be with someone close. In some the desire is clear and strong, in others less visible. Often the latter ones do not show such strong efforts in this direction, because due to their social roots, professional work, contact with colleagues, or own fantasies they do not feel their loneliness in an acute way. The schizophrenic feels it constantly.

## Communication with the Patient and the Intensity of Delusions

When talking to the psychotic person, we will grasp the meaning of his expressions only if, at the very beginning, we admit that what he experiences is meaningful, that he wants to express something important for him. We must accept that this man is exposed to and cannot cope with the issues that to some extent concern us, too, even if they do not disorganize our behavior. If we start from the recognition of the importance of his experiences, we will not focus on words that will seem so senseless. We will then be able to lead to a compromise and make the patient's speech closer to generally accepted meanings. When such a patient feels that we understand him, he will often follow us and begin to use a less psychotic way of expressing himself. So he will be recovering in this relationship.

If we detect the point of maximum emotional involvement of the patient, that is, if we bring his speech about politics, history, religion or secret experiments to the basic emotional problem, a surprising "recovery" may happen. The man will begin to get rid of part of his autism, talk about his grief and sorrow, about the father or mother, with enthusiasm, sometimes with tears.

When in turn there is no empathy and the ability to find meanings, the patient will become overwhelmed by more and more "senseless" concepts and statements. The force of the delusion, so assertion, with which it is presented, often depends on the nature of the relation between the doctor and the patient. This indicates the importance of the pragmatic, communicational aspect of the delusion, in contrast to the purely semantic aspect. The quality of the relationship has an impact on the level of psychological integration and presented symptoms (Jarosz 2000, 766).

This is illustrated by an event that took place when I went with a schizophrenic patient, Robert, to the so-called "school of life," where he, after several months of stay in the hospital, was supposed to undertake occupational therapy. We talked on the way, and Robert was logical and interactive, although obviously frightened and lost in the new situation. It seemed that the form of "school of life" would be more appropriate for his rehabilitation than a further stay in the hospital. However, considering the drawbacks of the monotonous stay in the hospital ward, I did not take into account the positive factor, which was the sense of security. Although I did not conduct Robert's systematic psychotherapy, during his six-month stay in the ward I met him and talked to him many times. Our meetings passed through various phases; sometimes Robert approached me, and sometimes he insulted me. I tolerated it, and although I was often tired of him, I tried to understand and not reject him. It was the same with other personnel members, who became familiar to him during these months of his stay in the ward. Robert went through a lot, and we went through a lot with him, which made him stop fearing us and become capable of intersubjective communication.

On arrival, in front of the office of the local psychiatrist, Robert started saying more and more things that were incomprehensible to me. When he was inside, it got even worse. The psychiatrist clearly had no patience for another "psychotic." Bored with her profession, she was almost openly aggressive. Robert could feel the atmosphere of this relationship, and because he was not yet strong enough to ignore it, he plunged into gibberish, abstract words.

What happened? The answer is that since the doctor was distant, he also grew away internally and abandoned the intelligible communication. At the end the psychiatrist said, as if to herself: "He will not stay here long." Robert did not let her down, he became "insane" again and was soon transferred to the ward.

The described situation indicates the obvious, yet overlooked, fact that speech takes place in a relationship and that it does not just name some objects but it leads to empathy, mutual agreement of actions and observations.[30] The world of human relations is for the psyche as such more important than the world of objects. In the example above the psychiatrist—by her questions, psychiatric anamnesis—made the patient refer to an objective, social reality. But in her office reality was pure abstraction. She denied the truer reality. She, in a really "schizophrenic" way, made Robert not see and not react to her lack of interest, alienation, and aggressive fatalism towards him. But it was this reality that reached him most, and his response was a reaction to it. From a certain perspective it was quite an adequate response.

## The Structure of Delusions of Influence

The psychiatrist will at least assume schizophrenic psychosis if the patient's speech shows that he feels outside influence or access to the patient's psychic experiences and thoughts. Speaking about such sensations is almost a leitmotif of schizophrenia. Patients say that other people influence their minds from a distance, they read their thoughts, change them and insert their own. They feel that others manipulate their minds in various ways, using hypnosis, telepathy, or radio transmission. They have the impression that they melt, lose control over themselves, and that their minds gradually cease to belong to them. They think that everyone knows their thoughts, having direct access to them, as if their minds were a wave extended in space.

In order to analyze this issue, let us use a specific case. The patient in her fifties, a nice woman fully capable of interactive contact with people, claimed that her mother sent thoughts to her and "sat in her." This woman was heavily influenced by her mother for the whole life, and was not allowed to be self-reliant. The mother was a selfish person, aiming to constantly control the daughter. She interfered in her daughter's marriage and did not accept her husband. After he left, she undermined her parental competences and tried to take over the care and control of her children. The patient said, "She (the mother) would like the children, grandchildren, and she would sit on it, then she would be happy"; "What did she do with me, she grinded me down"; "She takes care of herself, she will outlive us all." She also said that "the mother does not know some of the words," "does not know what ass, cunt, cocksucker mean, she says that a man has a sock between his legs." The mother purportedly "sat in the lips" of her daughter, willing to learn these words from her. According to the daughter, she was "perverted" and "stood out from the norm."

Can we, based on these statements, understand more than that they point to the mother-daughter conflict and relate to sexuality? Let us take a closer look. The mother demonstrates sexual ignorance, she has, among other things, the wrong idea about the male genitals. We can say that this ignorance refers to male-female sexual activity in general. The daughter has this knowledge. The mother enters the daughter, without her consent, and tries to take advantage of this knowledge. To put it simply: the mother wants to live her daughter's sexual life. This type of desire occurs quite often in mother-daughter relationships, in which the mother does not allow the daughter's autonomy as a woman and a person. They may occur between a mother and her anorexic daughter, a daughter with a personality disorder, a neurotic daughter. They can manifest themselves in thousands of ways, and are often almost impossible to notice without analysis in psychotherapy. Such patterns may also concern relations where the daughter does not suffer from clinical disorders.

Jung wrote about the archetypal aspect of the mythological Demeter and Kore, mother and daughter, who:

> extend the feminine consciousness both upwards and downwards. They add an "older and younger," "stronger and weaker" dimension to it and widen out the narrowly limited conscious mind bound in space and time, giving it intimations of a greater and more comprehensive personality which has a share in the eternal course of things. [. . .] We could therefore say that every mother contains her daughter in herself and every daughter her mother, and that every woman extends backwards into her mother and forwards into her daughter. [. . .] The conscious experience of these ties produces the feeling that her life is spread out over generations—the first step towards the immediate experience and conviction of being outside time, which brings with it a feeling of *immortality.* (Jung 1980, 188)

Manifestation of this archetype can take a negative form if—instead of being a way to broaden the consciousness—it is put directly into practice. The mother's interference in the daughter's emerging or already shaped sexuality (femininity) can be a kind of living the daughter's life. Such a situation arises when the mother cannot cope with the fact that the child is a separate being, keeping the child at the pole of dependence. She is afraid of the contact with her daughter as an autonomous person, having her own needs and relationships (the relationship with her father, which is independent of the mother's relationship with this man, is the prototype here). Then the development of the relationship is not going from the original resonance towards the dialogue, but the "face-to-face" contact is permanently replaced with entanglement. The arisen situation is highly pathogenic, although it can look otherwise from the outside. Although the mother does not simply reject the daughter, she rejects her individuality and autonomy. As grandmothers, such mothers may undermine the parenting competences of their daughters, because they do not fully recognize the fact of their femininity. They try to obtain the maximum impact on the upbringing of their grandchild, which can border on taking the child away from its mother (they may constantly complain that the grandchild "looks bad," is "undernourished" and "nervous"). As a result of rejection of the daughter's separateness, the mother does not accept the fact that the grandchild is a fruit of an intimate and exclusive meeting of her daughter with a man. Without feeling obvious boundaries between herself and her daughter, she functions as if she were impregnated and gave birth herself. Such an unconscious illusion may arise because the mother wants to see only herself as a real woman and fully a person, the daughter is supposed to remain a child, actually someone with no individuality.

Beside sexual impulses, we see the fear of death behind the mother's behaviors. The defense against it takes place according to the following scheme: "If I am a woman and my daughter is just a child, I am still young, I will not die yet." To elucidate this a little closer, let us use the patient's other statements: "Mother says to me in my head that no one will entomb her, that she will outlive everyone; another mother has ten children and goes to the grave, she does not stick to any of them; it is unbelievable to treat one's diseases with children; she treats cancer with me; she was supposed not to walk, but she would still jump over you; she sits in my eyes, lips, teeth; she broke all my teeth."

What do we deal with in this case? This is a description of some psychotic interpersonal reality. It is about the mother unable to accept the natural way of life and death, about the mother undermining the daughter's life forces. Here we deal with a behavior destroying the vitality of the child and the desire to live longer than her. The daughter's psychotic state is a hallmark of the mother's pathology—it is the "delusions" that reveal the truth about their relationship, which in a normal state would never be verbalized. This kind of situation occurs in the case of mothers whose constant complaining about their health causes the feeling in the child that she is responsible for her mother's life. The message is clear: "You should (it usually concerns daughters) feel guilty that you will live longer." And indeed, I knew patients who, escaping the guilt, wanted to die first.

In most cases in which we deal with a dependent daughter tied with a sense of loyalty, the daughter who did not start a family or, despite having it, is focused on the mother most, we will discover the mother's pathological fear of old age and death. Such mothers cannot enjoy the daughter's independent life (sometimes they say: "What's the point in having you? I've raised you, and now you'll leave me") because her departure from home reminds them of the inevitable passage of time, of the generational change. Not wanting to let this happen, they mutilate their daughters, they make them emotionally and socially disabled. In this way, they avoid the succession of generations, because the mother is still the only real woman, the daughter is still an incomplete being, actually a child.

A more camouflaged form of the described situation, but with similar causes and consequences, is that when the mother is excessively worried about her child (often already grown-up). She keeps repeating that she is so worried about her child that her health breaks down. Such a mother's child withdraws her vitality, she stops going towards the world so as not to upset her mother. She is constantly thinking about the mother's condition, her health and life, and therefore gives up her own life. In this way, the mother somehow "does not let" the child live, "protects" her from old age and death, and therefore she "does not age" herself.

## Perception and Definition

The source of many psychotic experiences are mental areas that elude the control of the subject in a specific way. Let us consider the case of the patient we will call Caroline. She was a twenty-year-old student who developed the psychotic process a few months earlier (it was actually a border of psychosis, and her case did not fit any nosological entity). Caroline expressed delusional opinions (claimed, inter alia, that she was "dying"), but she remained in a logical contact, and in the course of sessions one could exactly understand the meaning of her experiences.

Caroline was always a "good child." She got the best marks at school, never caused problems for her parents. She was serious and responsible, genuinely interested in education and books. Fun, contact with her mother or father, seemed to be less important for her. However, her independence and achievements, and perhaps also intellectual capabilities became one of the first steps to the disease. How is it possible? We can say that at that time Caroline was "defined" as "calm-interested-in-learning-not-expecting-intimacy-good-pupil" by her parents, and mostly the mother, and then she was perceived only like this. Previously, the child probably lacked closeness with her mother. However, as well-developed intellectually, she coped with it herself, organizing her own world and partly isolating herself. If Caroline had been less talented, perhaps she would have demanded her mother's love more insistently. And perhaps the mother would have responded to her needs.

But when Caroline as a child enters primary school, she hides the deficit of emotional contact with her mother deep, which helps to distance from her. Because she is agile intellectually and does not cause any trouble to her parents, nobody pays attention to her. But what did the mentioned *defining* lead to in her life? Understanding this is a key that will allow to capture the genesis of the schizophrenic feeling of emptiness and to better comprehend identity disorders, and even delusions (impressions) of the mind being read.

Let us examine fragments of a family psychotherapeutic session, which was attended by Caroline and her mother. At the beginning of the meeting I asked the mother how she saw what was going on with her daughter. The mother began with the following words: "Caroline was always a very well-mannered girl." She continued with a description of Caroline's levels of education up to the period in which she no longer managed at the university. Only after a long speech there was a kind of the second stage: the mother said a little about the relationship of Caroline and her sister, about Caroline's isolation from her father at puberty, etc. Here are the next fragments of this session.

*Caroline*: "Mama doesn't understand it, but I'm really dying" (with a shy smile on her face).

*Therapist*: "Why are you smiling, saying this?"

*Caroline*: "Well, because she doesn't believe me. She thinks that everything will be okay, and I am dying. I don't exist anymore, I feel that my brain is eaten up, I don't feel anything inside. I'm dying and I'm afraid of it. Once, I wanted to die, and now I'm really scared. It'll start with the head, I don't know what will happen to my body, all the organs will stop working."

*Therapist*: "You feel that you're dying emotionally, that your mind is dying. You can't know what's happening to your physiology, but you feel that your psyche is dying."

*Caroline*: "Yes."

Caroline says that she "feels nothing," in fact, in a "blocked" way, she feels with all herself. The mother is actually sitting without expressing any emotions. The daughter, however, cannot accept this, because it is too painful, so she takes on the deadness of their relationship. Later in the session, I ask the mother and daughter to sit directly opposite each other. I want to provoke them into a more direct contact.

*Therapist*: "How do you feel now, Caroline?"

*Caroline*: (trembling a little): "I'm scared."

*Therapist*: "What would you like to tell your mom? Say it."

*Caroline*: "She should understand that I'm dying, it isn't a joke."

*Therapist*: "Caroline, don't say it to me, say it to your mom."

*Caroline*: "Mom, I'm dying, I'm getting weaker, and you don't believe me. Believe me, it won't be fine. I want to go to the sea and die there. You always say that I will recover, but I will not, mom. I exaggerated with this last time." (She is talking about taking amphetamine, which she believes is the cause of her present condition). "I didn't think about you, and now my brain stops working, I don't know how many cells I still have. Why did I do it, I could have not taken these drugs any longer, but I did. I wanted to die. You said to me: 'Well, you'll do it, and have you thought how we'd feel?' And I wasn't thinking about you, I ruined the family. I don't want to hurt you" (close to tears).

*Therapist*: "I think, Caroline, that you're afraid, too, that the family's grief after your death will be too small."

*Caroline*: (after a moment, softly): "I think this too."

Throughout all this sequence, the mother is silent. I feel that it lasts far too long, if this was not because of serious communication barriers between her and the daughter. I do not think about Caroline's mother as a "cold" or "bad" person, she is rather blocked. Leaning in the direction of Caroline, she is frowning, as if to intervene, but she does nothing. I think she lacks the "channel" that would allow her to emotionally communicate with her daughter. Not surprisingly, over the years, she referred only to "a well-mannered-student," and now her daughter showed the mysterious and untamed level of her emotional life.[31]

Caroline asked several times whether the brain cells may die, because she feels that "here"—she pointed at the parieto-occipital part of the head—she has "everything dead." I asked her what there was in that part of the brain that died in her opinion, what functions, what emotions. She said creativity, because she used to write poems and stories, and now she does not even remember what she just read. She said: "I have only the basic functions; I see, I hear, but I do not feel my body, I do not think with the whole head." I asked her to perform a simple exercise, to close her eyes. She immediately felt that she had to open them, that she could not stand it. She felt that this place on the head "pulls up" and "wants" her to open her eyes.

The top of the head represents the identity of Caroline as "a good pupil." She feels that it must be active twenty-four hours a day, that it cannot fall asleep (it "pulls up," provokes opening the eyes). When this part ceases to function, she will "die." Why? Because the remaining part of the brain will not work (in the therapeutic dialogue I say that she is "asleep" and not that she "died" to bring Caroline's language closer to the normal one). This part represents the sphere of personality, which was not accepted by the parents and remained unstructured. Caroline feels that her identity up to this time ("top of the head") breaks down and she does not know any other way of life (she cannot think with any other "part of the brain"). Therefore, she is scared of "death." Her fears are then reasonable—beyond the sphere of *definition* there is nothing that she could consider as her own, as herself, so this is an area of emptiness and death. The following dialogue completes it:

> *Caroline*: "I feel that when the conscious part on the top of my head gets tired and stops working, I'll die."
>
> *Therapist*: "Because you don't believe that the other part will wake up. It dreams a dream that you're a child, close to mom."

Caroline's dream had a similar meaning: "I'm sitting on the roof of a high-rise building, there are lots of people on the ground, I can't see them clearly. I fear that I'll fall. The skyscraper is narrow like a pole." In the dream, she also had a feeling that whichever side she tilted to, she would fall. Interpretation: Caroline is sitting on the top of the skyscraper, so in a very insecure place. This place is a symbol of her identity, it is the same as "the top of the head." The indistinct mass of people on the ground is the remaining sphere of her personality. It is chaotic and confusing, but as it is located at the base it can ensure stability. (Caroline: "they can't fall.")

To be, one has to be perceived. This sentence is not a rhetorical figure embellishing the text, but the statement, the meaning of which is manifested by clinical facts. A child for its proper development must be *perceived* by its parents.[32] That is what Caroline was missing. Caroline was not seen in her emotionality, weakness, childishness. The mother's eyes got stuck on the surface, at Caroline as "a good and well-mannered girl." The fantasies of her childhood are evidence of this deficit. When she went to primary school, she imagined that in one of the windows there was a man constantly watching her. He knew her every gesture, thought, feeling, and desire. He was reportedly an older, experienced man who was watching her with binoculars. She liked it, she appreciated that someone had interest in her.

I would like to once again emphasize this point: *perception* in the parent-child relationship has the power of formation. It is more than just perception understood commonly—what is unnoticed in a child will not develop, will develop defective or will become so vague that the child will not be able to manage with it.

To illustrate this, let us take an example of another girl. Although she did not demonstrate a psychotic disorder, she had serious problems in interpersonal relations, in organizing her life. She had strange feelings and did not feel well with herself. Like Caroline, she took care of herself in her childhood. She played by herself, learned without help, did not cause problems. Today she is mentally dependent on her parents, who never paid enough attention to her. She unwittingly destroys everything that could lead her to adulthood, that is her studies, mature relationships, and even psychotherapy, as being independent is accompanied by a huge fear of the ultimate loss of her parents.

The girl told me that whenever she did anything, and the parents appeared near her, she started doing something else. I understand it this way that she could not show them even a scrap of her spontaneity—only the action started with the arrival of the parents was created enough to be seen by them. In her early childhood the girl must have felt that it was better to give up her spontaneity, and to maintain the acceptance of the parents she learned to pretend. The parents not only did not show enough attention, but always had the same point of view (the patient considered them as "one"), which was hard for her. A certain degree of divergence and complementarity of opinions is advantageous, for each of the parents may see the aspect of the child's personality unnoticed by the other one. In this case, this was missing.

What is characteristic in her experience is the specific response to the gaze of others. If someone watched her for a while, he became "eliminated," it was not possible for her to familiarize with such a person. When someone watches her, she feels insecure. As if she were afraid that the stranger will notice something that she does not know herself, and this way he will have the knowledge that she lacks. And that would be a kind of appropriation of her person. Looking at her he would do what the parents were supposed to do—see the aspects that she cannot hide and control, that are not processed by the play, gesture, and mask. She could not let that happen, because the stranger would probably do it without appropriate attention and love. Thus, he would only stimulate her hidden pain. So we see that in her response to the gaze of another person, in a camouflaged way, her longing for the look of the parents returned.

Not *perceiving* the child stops the structuring of certain aspects of its personality. What is constituted only in the relationship, not being taken up by parents, remains in the stage of undifferentiation. The so-called overprotection is probably the most common method to avoid perceiving the child. This attitude is common in mothers, less available to fathers. In its course a projection of own narcissism to a child is quite frequent (Freud 1957b, 90–91), and the child becomes an ideal being to the parent. The parent does not acknowledge that the child is imperfect, sexual as well as aggressive and mortal. The parents want to see in the child what they will never become themselves, deny the passage of time, transience, and imperfection of the world thanks to the child. The child must make all their secret dreams come true, even those totally unrealistic. Guided by these desires, they avoid seeing the truth about their child, they basically negate his or her existence as a human being, wishing him or her to be the ideal them. Everything that denies the idealized image irritates them and is rejected.

With this attitude, the parents live an illusion, and their contact with the child is shallow. The child, in turn, quickly learns to hide the unacceptable aspects of itself, which in the future may become the cause of its problems, including an identity crisis. By her attitude the mother controls and seizes the child, and although apparently the child is in the center of interest, in fact, the mother is the central figure. She always knows best what her child needs, and therefore she does not actually have to listen to him or her. The child becomes her extension, and not an independent being. The mother gives the child everything so that he or she does not begin to talk about his or her needs. She does not want to hear this, because she is afraid of the fact that a separate person is growing next to her. Therefore, she "neutralizes" the independence and individuality of the child by making the child dependent on her.

This attitude is not much different from the explicit rejection, because the mother takes care of the child and loves him or her so far as he or she is dependent on her. But she rejects the child as someone for themselves. She rejects the "inside" of the child, that is, his or her subjectivity, affirming at most his or her "externality," that is, what she wants the child to be.

## Perception in Psychotherapy and in the Family

The importance of perception is also proved by insight psychotherapy. While in the process of psychotherapy, the patient should feel that he is accepted by the psychotherapist, or even receive a certain amount of love, it is obvious that the level of warm feelings the therapist can give does not fill the emotional holes of most of the treated people. The therapist can devote more time to the patient and give him more and more warmth, becoming his substitutive and also a better parent, but such an attitude usually leads astray. The level of care will still be insufficient for the patient, and he will begin to increase his demands and expectations. Such a situation can lead to an adverse effect—the therapist, instead of filling his patient's emotional gaps, will provide him with another disappointment. Simply, no longer able to stand the escalating demands, the frustrated therapist will reject him as wayward and ungrateful. The therapist, who happened to experience such a situation, did not take into account the fact that being a true parent is associated with emotional sacrifices and input we would not be able to offer to anyone, except for our own children. So in some sense, this therapist—even though he meant well—cheated his patient.

The therapist, even without sacrifice and strenuous emotional investment, can give a lot. In addition to, as we have said, the limited pool of compassion, love, and desire to help, he can offer something that will heal the wounds that the parental love did not. That something is the perception included in the interpretation. Interpretation makes it possible to ease extreme emotions, get rid of the physical pain, distance from despair. When we cannot capture the patient's experience in a correct interpretation, he may at some point not withstand, leave, drop out of the therapy or even go berserk. When we capture it, the patient calms down, has a sense of closeness. Why does it happen? It is not that the patient deliberately wants to tell us something, and becomes angry because we do not understand it. We can understand what he says to us, we can respond with our understanding, and he can confirm it. And despite this he will not stand it, he will feel irritated, angry, helpless, and misunderstood. The therapist's goal is to catch what the patient has "on the tip of the tongue," but what he will never see and express without help. This unconscious tortures and enslaves him. When spotted, the patient feels integration. (I disregard here the aspect of resistance against the consciousness and the discomfort resulting from it—we ease the resistance also through interpretation.)

A similar mechanism occurs in the case of a relationship between the parent and child. The parent should see what happens and forms in the child. The parent should give space for expression and field for structuring of what emerges and what the child does not understand yet. This applies, for example, to aggression, sexuality, fears, weaknesses. The parents cannot pretend not to see these aspects of the child's personality. They cannot leave them on their own, or excessively control and smother them. They must be able to observe and try to understand them. Otherwise, the child will get the message: "do not develop this," "be ashamed of this" or "destroy it!" And it is a matter of the most vital aspects of the personality. The structure of the child's psyche forms in relationships, and it is the nature of the relationship with parents that makes creating the compact *self* possible, or causes that a stable identity will never be born. The psyche only to a limited extent develops "by itself," based on the genetic program.[33] The child grows physically, becomes more and more skillful manually, speaks better and better, knows more and more. Everything looks very promising. The child is healthy and capable intellectually, he or she learns well and is "polite." But at the same time the child's personal-emotional structure can develop into adverse directions. A symbiotic, self-mutilated person can come into being, a person who will be dependent in the future, with a deeply hidden palette of negative emotions.

Psychotics were not sufficiently "consolidated" as individuals in the course of their relationships with the guardians in childhood. That is why they remain specifically dependent on relationships, they can strengthen or crush them, which is manifested by delusions of mind being read and external control. To avoid a complete breakdown, they enter a phase of detachment from the social world, autism. Then it is very difficult to make contact with them. The paradox of schizophrenia is that it has the aspect of extreme sensitivity to relationships and—at the same time—extreme indifference to them.

## COURT AND GOD—CLINICAL CASE STUDY

Dominica, in her thirties, was a psychologist, and her life was filled with legal disputes and cases in court—against the employers who dismissed her, against the personnel in the hospital she was generally dissatisfied with, against the lawyers who—in her opinion—failed to run her cases properly, against the witnesses who did not testify what she wanted to hear and even with the judges, who were "biased." In some respects she was quite efficient in life, for example, after each dismissal she could find herself another job, but in other areas, she was completely disorganized. The latter concerned mainly her relationships with people. For years, even though she lived alone, she remained in contact with aid and care institutions, visiting psychiatrists and various centers. She never went through real psychotherapy, she interrupted the ones she had started or entered into rather loose and unstructured contacts. During her stay in the psychiatric ward, where I worked, she was aggressive and loud, with a great ability to cause resentment or even fear in the staff members.

Although the patient did not display positive symptoms, or any other symptoms of clinical psychosis, the analysis of her biography and functioning leaves no doubt that she was a psychotic person, in the sense of the psychotic personality structure (she fulfilled the criteria for what was once referred to as "litigious paranoia").

Dominica never felt that she was fully "in her body." As though she had not been where she was seen. Instead, there was something that she felt above her, something that watched her actions from a distance. This *quasi-observer* was associated with the law, the courts, and with what is social and supraindividual.

Dominica's functioning was characteristic. In relations with people, she invariably provoked conflicts with her demanding attitude, continuous dissatisfaction, and endless claims. Although she was an educated and intelligent person, she often acted as if she did not understand the basic principles of coexistence with people. She complained about her undue responsibility and the compulsion to remain "good-mannered." She tried to make friends with her doctors, at the same time wanting them to keep the professional attitude, which she *nota bene* constantly criticized.

When she stopped the therapy, she wanted me to be her friend, but she still expected "therapeutic" understanding. From the people around she expected care as a child, but she did not express this desire in the form of a child's request at all, it was rather a "parent's" demand. She reacted strongly to "harm" (and real harm), which other patients experienced in the hospital, but eventually she always referred to her own grievances. Although she felt internally weak, in need of support, and perhaps she even cried, on the outside she was always teasing and criticizing, with a raised voice. All this contributed to a conglomerate of behaviors difficult for the observer to decode, and the inconsistency of her attitude drove to constant conflicts. Other people were not able to understand her, nor could they adequately respond to her messages.

It seems that writing complaints and lawsuits was one of Dominica's basic ways of life. It is characteristic that she did not care about the final result as much as she did about the kind of dialogue with the defendant. She called it the "silent dialogue"—she obtained satisfaction, regardless of the fact that the case was fought in absentia and without personal contact of the parties. Dominica could not give up filing suits. She needed court in order to be able to enter into any dialogue with people. Without the realm of the law she felt isolated, lonely and worthless.

Why did this happen? We can say that in contact with another person Dominica "did not treat herself seriously," and because of this she treated another person in an "unserious way" too. At the same time she belittled the importance of the contact itself. This should be understood properly. The point is that Dominica in a sense *did not feel* that her existence as a person happened "here and now," that she was a psycho-physical being in contact with another, equal being. She had the impression that because the important "part" of her person was somewhere "above," therefore, what happened "down below" meant little (these are my own definitions, created on the basis of what the patient said). That is why she could not dispose of the feeling that such a conversation did not make much sense, that the "face-to-face" contact was just a mask, and the meeting was not possible, because what was most important for her was somewhere on the side or above her.

This attitude was a source of conflicts, as Dominica, faulting people and uttering opinions, was to some extent absent at the same time. She could complete the meeting only through the court system. In her life, the law and the courts were not what they are for an average man. They did not play a purely practical role, but had a psychological meaning. Anyway, she was never satisfied with the result of the cases. It was never what she meant, the way she wanted it to happen, it was never enough.

To understand this we need to capture the basic feature of her psyche. I would say that the woman was absorbed in the *universal* sphere much more than an average person, and neglected the *individual* one. Living as a person, as "an empirical being," she did not feel satisfaction and fullness of life. Her existence was completed somewhere "above" herself. Her "higher" part could be fulfilled and express itself only in the supraindividual sphere. This sphere was constituted and maintained by the letter of law and the court procedure. She paid much attention to official papers and national symbols, although she wrote her letters carelessly and messily. She demanded the seriousness of the institution and claimed that the judges did not behave in an appropriate way, but she did not respond to the judges' requests, and she even used vulgarisms.

The legal and public sphere gave her temporary peace and a sense of security resulting from the contact with something higher and pervasive, beyond a single man. Dominica's litigiousness resulted from a specific fixation on the area. Dominica turned to this direction, because she saw something repulsive and perhaps frightening in the individual aspect of her existence. Interpersonal relations that were not mediated by the legal sphere were also not satisfactory for her. This was because her specific *quasi-observer* could not take part in them. That *observer* was a dissociated and a kind of "objectified" part of her *self*. It was possible for her to fully involve the *observer* in life, use it in a dialogue with the other only within as much "objective" judiciary and law.

How could this type of personality structure be formed? Of course, it is impossible to accurately reconstruct it, only some aspect of Dominica's upbringing may shed some light on the matter. When she was a child, her mother often spoke not directly to her, but impersonally. For example, she entered the room and said: "The window is open again, and father is so sensitive to drafts." It was clear that she blamed the girl and demanded to close the window, but did not say so explicitly. What did such a style of communication with the child include? First of all, annihilation of the direct relationship. Speaking this way, the mother reached all practical purposes (e.g., closing the window), could express her emotions (e.g., discontent) and criticism, and at the same time she did not enter a direct relationship with her daughter. In such a situation, the child could not really say anything because there was formally no conversation with the mother. The contact with the mother was then mediated by the sphere of general principles. We can imagine that taking up a "dialogue" with the mother would lead to equally impersonal statements.

One day, Dominica woke up at night and felt that she "is in herself." She thought then, to her surprise, that she could stop writing complaints. When she told me about this a few days later, she said, however, that she was afraid she would lose "this god" (this is how she began to define the transpersonal realm), that it was something "otherworldly." I asked her then about her attitude towards the "ordinary" God, about religion in her life. She replied that she felt sometimes the solemn atmosphere of the church, added two sentences, and soon afterwards referred to national ceremonies and court hearings. She admitted that for her "the god in court is bigger."

The creation of Dominica's "individual" god includes processes similar to those which Émile Durkheim pointed out in his concept of the genesis of religious feelings and ideas. Durkheim said that religion is man's attitude to the *sacred*, of course impossible without previous division of the world into the *sacred* and the *profane*. He posed the question, where the sacred sphere in human life comes from, and answered that the *sacred* derives from the social. Experiencing the *sacred* is thus a kind of "contact" with society. However, in Durkheim's concept, "society" is not only the name given to the human community, but something existing in reality. A supraindividual being, *Society*. It has its own autonomy and specific objectives.[34] *Society* understood this way emerges as a result of a synthesis of the individual consciousnesses, as a kind of "superconsciousness," which has its own rules and practices, a kind of "superthinking" that is categorial-conceptual and impersonally logic reasoning. Durkheim wrote: "If it [the concept] is common to all, it is the work of the community. Since it bears the mark of no particular mind, it is clear that it was elaborated by a unique intelligence, where all others meet each other, and after a fashion, come to nourish themselves" (Durkheim 2008, 434). And later:

> The collective consciousness is the highest form of the psychic life, since it is the consciousness of the consciousnesses. Being placed outside of and above individual and local contingencies, it sees things only in their permanent and essential aspects, which it crystallizes into communicable ideas. At the same time that it sees from above, it sees farther; at every moment of time, it embraces all known reality; that is why it alone can furnish the mind with the moulds which are applicable to the totality of things and which make it possible to think of them, (Durkheim 2008, 444)

Only participation in social mind protects an individual from chaos of the incommunicable subjectivity. It is *Society* that creates concepts, and thus logic reasoning, which in particular clearly applies to categories, so the most basic concepts (these include the concepts of time, space, type, number, material, causes, etc.). Durkheim argues that these concepts could not be formed in the mind of an individual, but they are "collective ideas," and that means they could be created only in the community. And what is important, categories not only originated in the community, they directly refer to it and express its states. We can say that within the categories, *Society* thinks about itself ("space" is originally the space of the group, "time"—the time of the group and subsequent generations, etc.).

The question of the existence of "two spheres" in human life is not new. It probably started with Plato's theory of ideas, it was then developed by Aristotle, and in the Middle Ages it took the form of the famous dispute over universals. The question is whether there are "general objects" or only individual objects; whether something in reality corresponds to general concepts (such as "table," "horse" or "man"), or if they are mere products of the mind. To simplify: is there any "horsehood," or are there only particular individuals, and the mind produces the concept of "horse" through abstraction? The legitimacy of this question is fully reinforced only by referring to mathematics: it seems that there must be an ideal circle, for example, a circle itself, and not only those imperfect "copies" that we are able to draw. So there is a question about the status of objects, the existence of which seems to be independent of particular, physical products (something like a computer program, for example).

The dispute over universals had broad implications, including religious ones, and the settlement is not obvious. I will not analyze it here, let me just indicate that this philosophical problem has an analogy in mental dynamics. We are interested in the psychological level, the meaning of the *universal* area to an individual psyche.[35] To relate all of this to the individual psyche, I will refer to Durkheim's reflections on the genesis of the concept of the soul. He started with the fact that the human soul has always been associated with the sphere of the *sacred*. And the *sacred* is a derivative of what is collective and social. So if there is something "holy" in man, it cannot be an individual factor, but an element transmitted to him by the group. The soul represents in us what is "different from ourselves," it was born from what is noble and moral, and only social life could make the individual accept this. What we call the soul seems to us something independent of the organic factor. According to Durkheim's concept, it is so because the soul is the representation of society within our personality. In other words, what we recognize in ourselves as the soul is a psychic instance constituted as result of introjection (internalization) of *Society*. Because this society—which is the source of ideas, moral feelings and higher mental activities—stands in opposition to the individual attributes of single man, and thus his senses, subjectivity and corporeality. Let us quote Durkheim again:

It is perfectly true that we are made up of two distinct parts, which are opposed to one another as the sacred to the profane, and we may say that, in a certain sense, there is divinity in us. For society, this unique source of all that is sacred, does not limit itself to moving us from without and affecting us for the moment; it establishes itself in us in a durable manner. It arouses within us a whole world of ideas and sentiments which express it but which, at the same time, form an integral and permanent part of ourselves. [. . .] Moral ideas have the same character. It is society which forces them upon us, and as the respect inspired by it is naturally extended to all that comes from it, its imperative rules of conduct are invested, by reason of their origin, with an authority and a dignity which is shared by none of our internal states. [. . .] In this voice which makes itself heard only to give us orders and establish prohibitions, we cannot recognize our own voices; the very tone in which it speaks to us warns us that it expresses something within us that is not of ourselves. This is the objective foundation of the idea of the soul: those representations whose flow constitutes our interior life are of two different species which are irreducible one into another. Some concern themselves with the external and material world; others, with an ideal world to which we attribute a moral superiority over the first. So we are really made up of two beings facing in different and almost contrary directions, one of whom exercises a real pre-eminence over the other. Such is the profound meaning of the antithesis which all men have more or less clearly conceived between the body and the soul, the material and the spiritual beings who coexist within us. [. . .] It remains true that our nature is double; there really is a particle of divinity in us because there is within us a particle of these great ideas which are the soul of the group. (Durkheim 2008, 262–63)

Durkheim says that man actually lives a double life: the life of an empirical, subjective individual, and the life of reason, ideas, generality and collectivity. This division applies to the very structure of the psyche, which splits into an individual and universal one. The universal sphere has a peculiar status: it is in me and opposes me at the same time, it represents something that is not me, something higher, "supernatural." The voice of this sphere is heard when it commands or forbids.[36] And this takes place mainly in court. Dominica's case shows that the division that Durkheim pointed to is the source of real mental dynamics and may have psychopathological consequences. At the same time, this case shows that, on the psychic level, "supernaturality," society, the universal sphere, and courts can indeed, in a way, combine into one.

## HEAVEN AND HELL—CLINICAL CASE STUDY

Anna was treated pharmacologically for schizophrenia for several years and decided to undertake psychotherapy at the age of twenty-two. She did not have any productive symptoms during this period, such as hallucinations or delusions, but her mood was severely depressed and she showed signs of autism. Anna's first psychotic episode happened during a class trip when she was eighteen. She began to hallucinate visually, it seemed to her that white crosses appeared on some of her classmates' foreheads. She believed those crosses meant "pure friendship." The vast majority of people had such crosses, but the cross of one of the boys seemed to flicker and disappear. To Anna's mind the boy was thinking about sex.

The world of psychosis was a world of sense and joy for Anna. When the disease started, she felt that everything around her gained significance. She wanted that state to last and at the same time was afraid that it could end, that is why she "concentrated in the mind" on experiencing it. In her opinion, this concentration had an impact on the development of the disease. She felt that "God is the solution to all problems." During her psychotic episodes, people seemed "good" and had "brotherly love" for one another, and it was much easier for her to sustain satisfying relationships with them. As a young artist, Anna particularly strongly experienced the process of painting pictures. She had the impression that the colors she chose were the most appropriate, that every line and splash, every brushstroke was exactly what she had designed. One could say that it seemed to her that she painted the best possible version of a given painting, she in a way substantialized its very idea. She felt that her artistic expression was complete, that she was spontaneous and free.

Anna spoke a lot since the beginning of psychotherapy, but I felt she did not need me there. So I sat and tried to reconstruct in myself the world of experiences that she described to me. After some time, I began to understand what she was talking about. There was nothing strange about it. After all, psychosis uses psychic structures that are universal equipment of every human being. In one of the sessions, I told her that I could empathize with what she felt. In this way I wanted to get closer to her and at the same time show that her experiencing also has a universal dimension, that it is accessible to other people. However, Anna did not react to my attempts to get closer through understanding.

Further therapy clearly showed Anna's need to be special and to have her own world only for herself. Anna suffered wishing to be understood and to communicate with another human being, but on the other hand she was afraid of it and she basked in her distinctness. During the therapy sessions Anna constantly returned to the subject of her attempts to "be natural." She referred to examples of other people, said that they could be "natural," that they had normal interpersonal relationships. She said several times that she could not "listen to others" and that she "did not notice" people, which was a problem for her. Someone was talking to her and she was thinking of something else, as if neither that person nor his words were able to draw her into a relation-ship. In such situations Anna talked about the "lack of love" and at the same time claimed that other people had love in them and were able to show it to one another. She was afraid that her mother would die, and it would not affect her. She cried when she said that. I pointed to it, saying that it was her true feelings, but she seemed not to accept it.

Although Anna felt "different" and lonely, and wanted to be like everyone else, there was another stream of experiences in her, whose course served Anna's mind to compensate for the sense of alienation. Her "distinctness," which was undoubtedly a source of anguish, also gave her the feeling of being someone better. It could not be otherwise, because the psyche, even split, can never dispose of its component parts, but only uses them in vari-ous forms—some explicitly and the other indirectly. In each of us, next to "pieces" of love, there are also "pieces" of hatred, next to altruism—there is selfishness, next to the feeling of inferiority—pride. If only one is visible, it means that the other one is inactive, undeveloped, suppressed, or it mani-fests itself in the most covert form.[37] Anna said, "I'd like to be able to think about myself," and in a sense she could not do it. On the other hand, she was constantly concerned only with herself. It is not easy to understand this and similar contradictions, but we must try, because only this way we can get closer to cognition of the human psyche that builds its functioning from them.

Anna reported that, on a cold winter day, she had carried full bags, her hands were cold, but she did not put on gloves. Another time, she carried a hot glass of tea that did not burn her at all. She returned to those seemingly trivial events several times. But these events were a confirmation of the exis-tence of her internal strength, a sign of power. Such experiencing of them was a manifestation of the same mechanisms that produce delusions of grandeur and mission during the exacerbation of the disease.

Anna also had specific negative feelings about looking in the mirror, and she felt particularly bad when someone saw that she looked in it. She had the impression that they perceived the abnormality of her looking. She expressed this abnormality with the words: "I look as if I were checking if I am still there." These feelings correspond with the phenomena observed in narcissism, in which one's appearance is never ignored (what I have called *a reduced feeling of existence* is also noticeable here). Whatever Anna did in the presence of other people, she always thought how it looked, or more accu-rately, how to make it look "natural." When at work, filling a kettle with wa-ter was enough for her to become stressed of thinking about every movement and of trying to do the intended activity in the most "natural" way. However, the greater the willingness to be "natural" was, the stranger and more un-natural her behavior became. Anna manifested increased self-observation and could not "just" participate in a relationship, because she constantly tried to look at herself from the side. She had the need to control the expression of herself into the surroundings, and perceiving her by others had to be designed by herself. The fact that others would create images of her frightened her, and it must have created the impression that their perceptions would tear her to shreds, from which she would no longer build her own identity.

Anna obsessively divided people into "pretty" and "ugly," she said she could not help it. She saw others as one-dimensional personalities, as "saints" or "bad ones." She could not associate with people, tolerating their internal diversity, the coexistence of what is good and what is bad. Being in the imaginary world of one-dimensional people, even if some of them are absolutely "bad," is safer than being with real people, that is, complex and multidimensional. She often talked about certain small gestures that were indicative of someone's "normality," "goodness" or "sainthood" (all these terms seemed to be to some extent interchangeable). She said that a friend of hers stroked a dog, smiled, started talking to her, and that everything was "so normal." People around her were not real people but images, icons of the ideal poles of "good" and "evil." The obsessive divisions of people into the "good" and "bad" sometimes intensified, and sometimes weakened, but they were always a defensive activity, a way of dealing with the unacceptable reality.

A few weeks after the prematurely ended psychotherapy, Anna was hospitalized again. Her experiencing again took on psychotic features, although the symptoms were less severe and she had a greater distance to her condition. The basic religious theme that occurred was the vision of being in hell, which corresponded with her depressive mood. It probably started on the day Anna walked into the room, where another patient listened to a Catholic mass broadcast on the radio. She imagined that it was a satanic mass, that Satan himself was close, and all patients were damned or devils. In hell, as she later explained her imagination, one can be "bad," "sin" (i.e., have sex), "do what people do in the toilet, but in public," "make love to all patients," one does not have to listen to anyone, one just wants to eat and sleep. Anna began to pray to Satan ("I thought that I gave my soul to him. It was like in *Faust*. Everything is nicer now, everything comes easy to me in the ward—sex, conversations"). However, she was constantly afraid that this state would end, that she would do something "wrong" and would punish herself. And indeed, one day she stabbed a fork in her hand.

It is characteristic that, to some extent, she actively created and sustained her imaginations. She was no longer as psychotic as she had been during the first hospitalization, and she was able to "choose" what was going to happen to her. She could no longer cope with her drives through negation, so she decided to create a place where her needs could be fully satisfied. "Hell" seemed to be the best place for this. Anna understood hell as a place where all repression and restrictions of the drive sphere could be abolished. Due to the lack of a moral reference, it gave her the opportunity to avoid feeling guilty. However, Anna's hell turned out to be insufficiently hermetic, so it could not protect her from guilt and the associated self-destructive tendencies.

In the period of remission of acute psychotic symptoms, Anna kept a diary. She read a fragment to me: "How wonderful it is when a soul talks with a soul, both free of the body. I'm looking for my soul so far, yet it is so close. I obscure it myself and hide it with my body, crush it under a flush, don't let it go out to the world." I asked what the "soul" is to her, she replied, "The soul—it's easy to draw, paint, watch pictures, write letters, learn, read poems; the body—nothing makes you happy, you see nothing, you understand nothing, you're dead. You can kick and beat the dead, he won't shout to God." She also said that "the soul is not in the body but in front of it (strength) or behind it (weakness)." We can be in the front, but we go behind it in every moment of doubt. The soul can come to the front only through the constant exercise of the body and pushing it. It needs to survive the arduous transition, "pushing through" the body. And the body is "sticky" and holds it tight. The body cannot "talk to" the souls of other people, as "it's dust, it's dead." Just like people do not talk to things.

What she expressed in the above words can be analyzed in two ways: through seeing its pathological aspect, or an existential and religious one. The pathological aspect becomes visible when we consider her words in the context of the presented model of schizoidism. Anna "crushes her soul under a flush" and does not allow it to enter the world, which can be understood, among other things, in the way that her inner *self* is suppressed by the facade one. Anna blushed in most social situations, because she constantly thought about how she was perceived. Because she did not have full control over this participating part of the *self*, she could never be sure of it. In her diary she wrote that her soul should always be "in front of" the body, never "behind" it. This could express the fact that we truly live only when our life is an expression of the pursuing of the inner, spontaneous *self* that is not suppressed by the dependent, participating part. But we can also look at Anna's words through the prism of religion and the universal human experience. Then they express a Gnostic experience. Anna felt the "body cage" more clearly than others, just like the Gnostics. She felt her isolation from other people and the world, her lonely soul's anxiety.

# NOTES

1. This is true to some extent for each disorder—we need to make a conceptual reconstruction of its structure. This reconstruction will always be one of the possible. If I emphasize it in this case, it is because "schizophrenia" is a diagnosis and a label that, in our society, greatly burdens the patient.

2. Fleck wrote: "The modern concept of disease entity, for example, is an outcome of precisely such a development and by no means the only logical possibility. As history shows, it is feasible to introduce completely different classifications of diseases. Furthermore, it is possible to dispense with the concept of a disease entity altogether, and to speak only of various patients and incidences" (Fleck 1979, 21). And then, on a specific case: "Siegel also recognized, in his own way, protozoa-like structures as the causative agent of syphilis. If his findings had had the appropriate influence and received a proper measure of publicity throughout the thought collective, the concept of syphilis would be different today. Some syphilis cases according to present-day nomenclature would then perhaps be regarded as related to variola and other diseases caused by inclusion bodies. Some other cases would be considered indicative of a constitutional disease in the strict sense of the term. Following the train of thought characterized by the 'carnal scourge' idea, still another, completely different set of concepts concerning infectious disease and disease entities would have arisen. Ultimately we would still have reached a harmonious system of knowledge even along this line, but it would differ radically from the current one" (Fleck 1979, 39).

3. In an attempt to single out schizophrenia, I rely on groups of symptoms distinguished by Bleuler and the category of primary symptoms introduced by Kurt Schneider. According to Schneider, the first-rank symptoms in schizophrenia include: thought echo; dialoguing and commenting voices; impression of the external impact on the state of carnal thinking, will, feelings and motives; thought broadcasting; delusional perceptions (Sadock and Sadock 2008, 156).

4. Wizel defined his patient's disorder as "underdeveloped schizophrenia" (Wizel 2001, 171) in a person with the "schizoid" type (Wizel 2001, 165). The category of "underdeveloped schizophrenia" introduced by him should be regarded as an attempt to capture the continuum between schizophrenia in the strict sense and less spectacular disorders. Thus, this approach is close to that I present below.

5. Quotation translated from Polish by Barbara Gąstoł.

6. Blaise Pascal wrote: "There are then a great number of truths, both of faith and of morality, which seem contradictory, and which all hold good together in a wonderful system. The source of all heresies is the exclusion of some of these truths" (Pascal 2018, 258).

7. It is now even a cultural norm, a matter often recognized as indisputable. Most of the movies, novels, comics are based on dissociation-idealizing structure of the "white characters" and "villains." In countless films, screenwriters and directors murder the latter, leaving no room for even a shadow of remorse or reflection from the "white." Everything is clear and simple, because "the villains" were deprived of the status of the people, they are only icons of evil. If we were to discuss the destructive influence of movies, the primary pathogenic factor seems to be not the presentation

of murder and rape as such, nor the direct apology of evil. This factor is precisely the cliché consisting of the certain victory of the "white," which, instead of educating, causes a kind of neutralization of the ethical side. Because thanks to splitting and idealization an artificial world is created, a world in which moral choices are too bright and too easy, so they basically do not exist. In fact, every person contains constructive and destructive tendencies and the irreconcilable contradictions. So he will never take one of the poles, which are pure abstraction. Only when he becomes aware of this, he may awaken the moral consciousness in himself.

8. Quotation translated from Polish by Barbara Gąstoł.

9. In order to better exemplify this process, let us look at depression. This disorder is often characterized by a complete inability to make any decisions. While in the store, the man is not able to decide whether to buy bread or rolls. Here we have a similar mechanism of creating "sphericity" to avoid the creation of any "resultant." Because the action in a given direction determines the human, thereby it condemns to conflicts with those who move in other directions. Of course, all this takes place within the psyche, and the display of these processes is merely sketchy. Generally, it is about a restoration of the archetypal unity and self-sufficiency. It does not matter that the man in depression expects support from others, his "self-sufficiency" takes place at other levels. Take self-blame, so characteristic in depression. The person tells us: "it is all my fault," says that he is "bad," "hopeless," that he is "angry with himself that it happened to him," he accuses and humiliates himself. He tries to clearly show that, if he is angry, "it is only with himself," if he nurses a grudge, "it is only against himself." These statements serve as isolation, the person creates an isolated area of self-sufficiency inside himself. To have all of him for himself, he obtrusively evaluates himself and thus protects against any assessment from the outside. Let us notice a kind of splitting here: if there is an accusation, there must be an accuser. To be able to accuse, the accuser must have a distance to the accused and be recognized as morally better. So if the person with depression shows himself as someone condemned in every respect, he suggests the existence of the accuser, who is able to keep distance in relation to any guilt, because he did not commit any misconduct himself. The more guilty the accused, the cleaner the accuser. Certainly, the person with depression tells us, and maybe also feels that he is all bad, as though there was no place for the accuser. The Gordian knot of depression is that the more the person blames himself, the seemingly less space is left for the area of the clean accuser, but at the same time the more we need to presume his existence. The accuser is deeply hidden, and the depressive identifies himself with him only in his deepest essence. There he does not accept even a shadow of criticism, he is free from all judgment and dictates laws himself. At this point he accuses absolutely everyone and everything, because he feels that his pain and rage will not be relieved. This structure of the *self* protects his specific kind of autonomy and self-determination. However, in the real world the depressive person is dependent and not self-reliant. Feuerbach noticed the similar in the religious attitude: "When they talk of their sinfulness, of their corruption, do they not at the same time talk of their essence, of the significance and reality of their individual selves? Is he who always inspects his faults and defects in the mirror less vain and self-satisfied than he who only thinks of his virtue and handsomeness?" (Feuerbach 1980, 18). "The essence" that Feuerbach refers to would be the accuser.

10. Besides, there is a category of borderline disorders ("borderline personality"), which are understood by many as the borderline of psychosis (Goldstein 1990, 15–16).

11. Laing's standpoint is the closest to this approach of course (Laing 2001). In a phenomenological way, Laing describes the structures and mechanisms of schizoid personality (that is, of the man without "mental illness") and schizophrenic personality (that is, the man with psychosis), pointing correlations between them. He seems to take into account what is universal for the whole schizophrenic spectrum—that is, common to various disorders from psychopathy to psychosis (mainly its prodromal and descending phases)—and possible to understand. I am of the same opinion, and my conceptualizations—even though arisen independently—are similar to Laing's concepts.

12. These criteria include the excessive sense of importance and uniqueness, haughtiness and arrogance, need for admiration as well as lack of empathy and exploitive approach to people (Fauman 1994, 379–80).

13. Freud saw self-observation as one of the main reasons for the distinction of the *superego* [German: Über-Ich], and combined it with the function of conscience, recognizing that observation is a prelude to judgment (Freud 1933, 86). Here, however, I will not use the term of *superego*, because I believe that the observing instance ("*quasi-external observer*") functions independently of the function of conscience and the ideal of the *ego*. Narcissism is a disorder in which the autonomy of self-observation manifests itself particularly visibly.

14. Quotation translated from Polish by Barbara Gąstoł.

15. This identification of the control over the image with the control over the person resembles the fears of primitive cultures that someone would have their photograph or portrait (Frazer 1965, 182–83).

16. Quotation translated from Polish by Barbara Gąstoł.

17. The desire for individuality and uniqueness observed in other narcissistic people is just the other side of the same coin. These people want what they do (who they are) to be "only theirs," they want it to be incomparable with what others do (who they are). While in the case described in the text it is about hiding behind the "perfect standard," this functioning is supposed to make observation impossible by hiding behind what is "completely unique." Both ways are supposed to eliminate what is accidental, spontaneous, "so-so," and thus discovering the truth about the man. Both serve to create an image.

18. Quotation translated from Polish by Barbara Gąstoł.

19. Solipsism—a philosophical term indicating the doctrine that explains reality based on the assertion that only I, the explaining subject, exist, and the rest of the world is not real.

20. Echolalia consists in automatic repetition of words, echopraxia of gestures, and echomimia of the facial expressions of another person.

21. Although the catalyst of delusions in older people is undoubtedly the degenerative process of the brain, there must also be a psychological mechanism to create the structure of such a compactness that a delusion has.

22. I will not concentrate on the complex and not entirely clear origin of such desires. Their roots are definitely in the Oedipus complex, the resulting sense of male inferiority, as well as hidden homosexual tendencies. Maybe it is about the desire of seeing what Freud described as the primal scene, that is, the parents' sexual intercourse. The man would seek his father's sexuality, which he sees as being superior to his own, and would strive to repeat and understand the painful "betrayal" he suffered from the mother.

23. See chapter 1.

24. Anorexics can admit that—in terms of the person they talk to—they are slim, but their subjective sense is closer to them.

25. Of course, constructivism does not omit this construct. The Oedipus complex has not only been "discovered," but also "constructed." It is not a description of reality itself, the "ontically real" process. Theoretically speaking, its conceptual reconstruction could look different.

26. It is about the theory of dopamine. Today, this theory, considered even at the purely neurophysiological level, is regarded to be incomplete (Frith and Cahill 2001, 50).

27. Fleck wrote: "The disciplined and even-tempered mood, persisting through many generations of a collective [in terms of scientists' "collective thinking"], produces the 'real image' in exactly the same way as the feverish mood produces a hallucination. In both cases switch of mood (switch of thought style) and switch of image proceed in parallel" (Fleck 1979, 180).

28. According to Fromm, the conscious is what is allowed by society (similarly, Nietzsche recognized the consciousness for what is shared and communicable, and ultimately common). The unconscious includes the whole spectrum of potential ways of living, feeling and perception of reality, inaccessible to man in a given social structure (Fromm 2000a, 172).

29. Pascal described what scares the schizophrenic in interpersonal relations with the following words: "For each Self is the enemy, and would like to be the tyrant of all others" (Pascal 2018, 127).

30. Here is what Laing writes: "The standard texts [diagnostic descriptions] contain the descriptions of the behavior of people in a behavioral field that includes the psychiatrist. The behavior of the patient is to some extent a function of the behavior of the psychiatrist in the same behavioral field. The standard psychiatric patient is a function of the standard psychiatrist, and of the standard mental hospital" (Laing 2001, 28).

31. We must remember that although the attitude of the mother is an important factor here, it has its conditions and roots. Both the external situation such as work, material conditions or the husband's attitude, as well as the mother's inner situation, that is, for example, her own experience with parents, may be important here. It is supported by the positive feedback between the mother and child—the child begins to modify his or her behavior, and thus reinforces the mother's attitude. That is why the child becomes very "independent," "calm," "avoids hugs," "plays alone."

32. The concept of *"perception"* and its function is close to the notion of *"Container-Contained"* by Wilfred Bion, and the concept of "mirroring" by Donald

Winnicott (see Hinshelwood 1991, 246–53). However, it was created independently and differs from both of these (by being used in relation to the phenomenon of the "unstructured" part of the *self*, and by connection to the theory of the constructivist status of knowledge).

33. Statistical studies of heredity often seem to indicate the contrary. Showing a hereditary factor, they suggest that the conditionings essential for development are innate. Studies of this type are not able, however, to take such subtle variables, as the described herein, into account. One of the psychological characteristics, strongly determined genetically is intelligence. However, two equally intelligent, untreated psychiatrically people can present, respectively, a compact or a clearly broken emotional-personality structure.

34. Durkheim was often criticized for allegedly unauthorized hypostatizing (Malinowski 1990, 135–36). It is obvious, however, that it is impossible not to grant society—since it is a system—a certain degree of autonomous existence that is independent of any individual human being. Even if Durkheim's approach is not very accurate, describing society and its impact on an individual, we cannot ignore the aspects he tried to show, defining society as a kind of autonomous mind. Since Durkheim understands society in this special way, to distinguish this concept from the colloquial meaning we will use italics (*society*).

35. One can mention Karl Raimund Popper's concept of "world 3." World 3 contains objectified knowledge, theories and general problems (world 1 is the physical world, and 2 is the mental one). Human psyche (world 2) "connects" (Popper's expression) to that world, develops in contact with it and, of course, enriches and modifies it. Popper says outright that "the self or the ego is anchored in world 3, and that it cannot exist without world 3" (Popper 2000, 129). Popper's theory, in its psychological layer (showing the nature of the relations between the ego and world 3), is underdeveloped, but we can say that the author's intentions are precisely to indicate that the general, universal, or ideal factor (in the sense of Plato's concept) plays a specific and structural role in the individual psychic life.

36. Durkheim's description of the internal pressure, and where he sees the source of that pressure, is, of course, the prefiguration of Freud's assertions on the function of sense of right and wrong in the *superego*. Durkheim assumes a similar, to that of Freud, model of formation of that instance, which can be expressed as follows: something "external" (society, parents) → internalization → something "half-internal" (a sense of right and wrong, mental representation of society), so something that being "inside" retains certain attributes of an "outside" thing (a kind of "strangeness," opposing the individual desires). The issue of mental instance, which is on the "borderline" between something internal and external, appears in Freud's concept of the *superego*, in my descriptions of the *quasi-observer*, and in Durkheim's theory I refer to. Looking broadly, all these conceptualizations explore the same phenomenon, the same area.

37. Basing on this type of complementarity is, in my opinion, the basic heuristic principle in explaining various structures and mechanisms of the psyche. Its "classic" use is Freud's recognition of neurosis as the "negative of perversion." Freud puts it this way: "Wherever any such impulse is found in the unconscious which can be

paired with a contrasting one, it can regularly be demonstrated that the latter, too, is effective. Every 'active' perversion is here accompanied by its passive counterpart. He who in the unconscious is an exhibitionist is at the same time a *voyeur*; he who suffers from sadistic feelings as a result of repression will also show another reinforcement of the symptoms from the source of masochistic tendencies" (Freud 1938, 575–76).

# Chapter Six

# Demonic Possession

## THE PHENOMENON OF POSSESSION

Possession is one of the most extraordinary phenomena known to psychopathology, and its uniqueness lies in the fact that it seems to be separate from it. The very name of this phenomenon (Latin *possessio*) and its historical connotations suggest that we do not deal here with one of the ordinary disorders—for these are to begin and end within the individual psyche—but with a *sui generis* event that involves interference of an external and autonomous being. Of course, despite the rare image that involves personality change, altered voice timbre, and even new cognitive or physical capabilities, psychiatry recognizes possession as a disorder. The *ICD-10* classification includes the code *F44.3 Trance and possession disorders* as a subcategory of dissociative disorders. The classification states that "in some instances the individual acts as if taken over by another personality, spirit, deity, or 'force'" (*ICD-10*, 135). However, unlike other disorders, possession is incorporated into a very broad cultural context. It is a phenomenon known for thousands of years, being an important element of many religions and beliefs.

The New Testament speaks a lot about the possessed, Jesus "drives out the demons" that are the reason for madness, mutism (aphonia, alalia), somnambulism (sleepwalking, lunatism), and epileptic seizures.[1] Cases of similarly understood possession are also known in other cultures, and what possesses is not always the devil. One can be possessed by another kind of "spiritual being." The Jewish tradition uses the term "dybbuk" (meaning "to cling") to describe a malicious spirit that, connecting with the soul of a living person, changes his personality (Unterman 2000, 77). A dybbuk may be a "naked soul" wandering without rest or reincarnation, and it may also be a demon that, entering a woman, makes her a witch. He is driven out through exorcisms. In modern Egypt, one can become possessed by a genie (see Üstün et al. 1999, 206–208), a morally ambivalent spiritual being of the ancient Arabic and Koranic tradition that remains between people and angels (Kościelniak 1999, 213 and 221). There are also accounts of being possessed by souls, both of the living and the dead. There are psychotherapists who, with the help of hypnosis and other practices, conduct a kind of "psychotherapy" of spirits, which reportedly connected with the body or the psyche of their patients (Prątnicka, 2007, Fiore 1995). In Japanese culture, there is the concept of *ikiryō*—a spirit that left the body of a living person, for example, during sleep (Iwicka 2017, 85 et seq.). The most frequent reason why such a ghost appears is a conflict with the person who becomes a victim of the *ikiryō*, whereby the man to whom the *ikiryō* belongs may be completely unaware of his activity. *Ikiryō* can possess and lead to death, but his long stay outside the body also weakens the person to whom it belongs, which can lead to his death too. We have a very interesting concept here that shows that the "unconscious connection" affects both persons.

Possessions are not always involuntary and not always negative. In shamanism, an archaic form of contact with the *sacred* and a method of healing, it is believed that the world is full of souls and spirits (Hoppál 2009). Shamans make mystical "journeys" in a trance to find the souls of the sick, because they believe that someone's problems may result from the loss of their soul. Sometimes, however, they themselves let ghosts enter their bodies. The Siberian shaman says:

> When I shamanize, I am possessed by the *ajami* [protective female spirit] and auxiliary spirits: they penetrate me like smoke or moisture. When the *ajami* is in me, it is she who speaks through my mouth and governs everything. (Quoted in Eliade 1994b, 83–84)[2]

Possession by spirits is the basis of the syncretic Haitian religion of Voodoo (Haitian Vodou), in which the faithful enter into a trance and are mastered by the *loa*, spiritual intermediaries between god and people. The haunting spirit can convey knowledge, as is the case with Hebrew *magides* (Hebrew "preacher"), that is, heavenly mentors who make contact with man through dreams, visions, automatic writing or speaking through his mouth (Unterman 2000, 166–67). In antiquity, it was obvious that oracles, such as the Pythia, prophesied thanks to the god, who filled them and spoke through them (Oświęcimski 1989, 126 et seq.). Similarly, contemporary spiritualists and channelers say that a medium is mastered by a spirit that can transmit relevant information (Chudziński 2013). Generally speaking, the belief in the possibility to contact an "outside" mind that can reveal the future, tell us about the past, advise us on important matters, or help to recover has existed since the dawn of human civilization.

Christian religions argue that possession cannot have positive effects. According to their interpretation, it is always something bad, because what possesses is of a destructive nature.[3] In Catholicism, it is absolutely a personal being, a fallen angel, Satan. In Protestantism, things are a bit different and the nature of the demon is understood in a few ways (Wink 1984). Some see him as a personality, and others see a personified chaos and emptiness, or even a kind of spirit that emerges from flawed and inhuman social and organizational systems—which resembles the esoteric concepts of thoughtforms or egregors as collective products of human minds that obtain some autonomy and secondarily affect people.

Catholic religion assumes several possibilities of devilish interactions (Amorth 1997, 30–32). These include: external inflicting physical suffering (for example, Padre Pio physically beaten by the devil), demonic oppression (various diseases and unfortunate life events attributed to the devil), diabolical obsession (paroxysmal and obsessive states, obsessive suicidal thoughts), demonic attacks (attacks on objects and animals), and the most spectacular— possession. According to the *Roman Ritual* [*Rituale Romanum*], the liturgical book of the Church dated 1614, a man can be considered possessed when his behavior involves three indicators: he periodically has supernatural physical strength, speaks or understands foreign languages of which he had no prior knowledge, and has knowledge of remote or hidden things (Amorth 1999, 227). The *Ritual,* approved by Pope John Paul II in 1998, underlines that these three groups of symptoms rarely occur together, and admits that these phenomena do not necessarily have to be caused by the devil (Fontelle 2004, 98). This Ritual places more emphasis on signals of aversive reactions to the Catholic symbols of the *sacred* (Fontelle 2004; Kocańda 2004, 210 et seq.; Madre 1999, 120–21).[4]

## A Theological, Psychopathological Problem or a Question about the *Conditio Humana*?

If we address the issue of possession from the psychological perspective, we must analyze the one that "possesses" ("demon," "devil") and the one who is "possessed" on the common plane. There are psychopathological phenomena very similar to those displayed by the possessed, but they are less spectacular and more frequent. Even some ordinary experiences are comparable to this, which in its dramatic form takes the image of possession. So it seems that they can be considered on a continuum ranging from everyday experiences, through well-known psychopathological phenomena, to possession. Such a perspective makes it possible to approach the problem of possession by deriving it from less complex phenomena. Investigating possession this way, we approach it from the quantitative side—we see it as a great intensity of the phenomena and mechanisms that occur also elsewhere. The continuum is indirectly indicated by exorcists, who are willing to recognize types of indirect demonic influences, where there is no specific response to the exorcism, and yet prayers and other "religious" activities lead to improvement (Madre 1999, 152–53). What the exorcist classifies as possession can begin with the phenomena well known to psychopathology, the intensity of which increases over time. Also, some obviously psychological symptoms—such as obsessions, irritability, anxiety, compulsive masturbation—are associated by them with the influence of Satan (Scanlan and Cirner 1999, 23, 56 et seq.). So Satan does not always possess, but often torments and causes problems well-known to medicine.

Let us list the symptoms and phenomena that occur during possession or demonic oppression (see Amorth 1999, 111–17; Amorth 2002, 63–64), and are known to psychiatry and psychotherapy: "alternative personality" (that takes the form of a "demon" in the case of an exorcism), amnesia for the attack (while the "secondary" personality knows about the normal one), sudden change in behavior or life preferences (a "normal person" shows abnormal behavior and interests), huge aggression in a "quiet" person, obsessive thoughts (also blasphemous), impulses (e.g., suicidal) coming "as if from the outside," pseudoparalysis and atony, hallucinations (voices, a sense of someone's presence, a sense of being touched). The phenomena known to parapsychology include telekinesis, precognition, telepathy, and manifestations of cryptomnesia in the form of "speaking an unknown language."

Reading the reports of exorcists or people who were "freed," we also notice the etiological processes common to many psychological problems and possession: the destructive impact of being rejected by close relatives, traumas in perinatal, infantile, Oedipal periods, and in adolescence (so in the critical moments of life), sexual abuse (Amorth 2002, 128; Amyot 2007). Also, there are therapeutic factors that are common for exorcism and psychotherapy: the positive effect of abreaction; regular meetings lasting for many years (symptoms subside, as in other disorders, gradually); the impact of the "human factor" (various effectiveness, despite the fact that all exorcists act "in the name of Christ"; Amorth 2002, 141; Morabito 2011, 170). This overlap and mutual penetration of typically psychopathological and "demonic" (i.e., atypical of psychopathology) issues proves the validity of establishing the continuum.

However, if we take the exorcists' accounts seriously (Rodewyk 1995; Siegmund 2004), we must admit that possession has also a different dimension, distant from what we recognize as familiar. It turns out to be a strange and frightening experience, it breaks the principle of the continuum, and overwhelms our intellect and emotions. The intensity of the phenomena that accompany possession, such as speaking an unlearned language, clairvoyance, psychic influence on others, knowledge of past and future events, unusual way of experiencing the *sacred*, and finally—if the accounts are reliable—levitations and materializations (Amorth 1997, 118 and 127), is so spectacular that it can introduce serious doubts about the possibility of scientific investigation of possession. As one can see, we deal here with something extraordinary. With something that surely fits the religious thinking with its category of "supernatural."

But do we really deal here with something supernatural? Even the most unusual phenomena were observed also in other contexts. People acquired, in hypnosis or even after a head injury, new—for example musical or mathematical—skills, referred to as savant syndrome (Padgett and Seaberg 2014). Even the famous patient of Josef Breuer, Anna O., in a state of hysterical dissociation wrote with her left hand, in English and in Roman printed letters (not in German and Gothic calligraphy), which probably would not have been so easy in a normal state (Freud and Breuer 2008, 31). Many of these phenomena seem almost impossible—where do, for example, additional abilities or information in a damaged brain come from? If we accept the—quite well-founded—hypothesis about the existence of the information field, it will be possible to explain these puzzles (Sheldrake 2009). It is worth knowing that telepathy and telekinesis have been tested experimentally, and the fact that there are still disputes about their existence is only a manifestation of the strength of the paradigm and the intellectual stiffness of the adversaries (McTaggart 2008, Cardeña 2018). The phenomenon of clairvoyance has been indisputably proved completely regardless of science—through the achievements of the Polish clairvoyant, Krzysztof Jackowski, who found hundreds of missing persons, helped to solve several criminal cases, and predicted many important world events (Jackowski and Janoszka 2018). There is evidence in the form of police certificates, films and texts published before the foreseen events, and even "live" recordings of successful clairvoyance sessions.

One of the tests to verify the presence of the "evil spirit" in a person is to give him holy water without his knowledge (Amorth 1999, 113). If the individual reacts aversively, it is supposed to be evidence of possession. The phenomenon is indeed surprising, it seems to indicate a real difference between ordinary water and holy water, and the sensitivity of the "evil spirit" to the latter. Is holy water truly "holy," since it has such power of influence? Franz Anton Mesmer, the author of the theory of animal magnetism, once made an experiment in which a woman immersed in a magnetic trance was touched sequentially with glasses of water. Only the glass he had touched before caused convulsions (Trillat 1993, 71). The water in this glass, although chemically unchanged, must have somehow distinguished itself from other waters, since it was recognizable. But is it possible? Was the water marked? This is quite possible considering the effect of homeopathy. In any case, the possessed person activates the extrasensory perception that is the equipment of every human being, but in normal states usually occurs sporadically in the form of intuition, empathy, or a prophetic dream. A greater cognitive challenge is levitation of the body, which has not been convincingly proven (Amorth and Sznurkowski 2017, 92), but lifting physical objects through mind power has been observed (Ostrzycka and Rymuszko 1989; Ostrzycka and Rymuszko 1994).

What happens to a possessed person is presented as completely foreign and inhuman. But is it really so? It may seem that the anger expressed by the "usually calm and nice person" during a possession crisis must be a sign of external interference. This is where, during the exorcism, this animal rage and inhuman screams come from. But maybe we should not judge this based on daily observation? In ordinary situations, none of us reveals the depths of our emotions and impulses, nor even experiences them. Psychotherapy uncovers the destructive impulses of ordinary people, and some therapeutic techniques directly expose internal "demons" through, for instance, provoking the expression of rage. The author of bioenergetics, Alexander Lowen, claimed that "a murderous rage seems to be present in every person who was beaten as a child" (Lowen 1997, 157). During therapeutic sessions, he made the patient burst into rage, which was expressed by screaming and pounding with fists or a tennis racket on the mattress. For an outside observer, this could seem frightening. If a person experiences regression, he may stop expressing himself with words and start shouting or howling. When he reaches the repressed and suppressed emotions of the early stages of life, he feels a natural need for nonverbal expression.

During sessions with the use of LSD, Grof observed that some people made strange facial expressions, gave the evil eye, started to vomit, or spoke in a changed voice. He describes a young woman whose problems and symptoms were particularly severe. She had suicidal tendencies, suffered from depression, she was a drug addict and alcoholic, she also suffered from painful facial cramps. Psychotropic drugs did not improve her condition. During one of the sessions, her facial cramps became unbearable, and finally her face took the form of a "mask of evil." The patient introduced herself in a changed voice as the "Devil." Grof felt something that seemed quite similar to my own feelings when I watched an attack of possession—the ominous atmosphere and the almost tangible presence of evil. The patient threatened the psychiatrist and she referred to the facts she could not possibly know about. Grof held her hand for two hours, imagining the bright light that the powers of darkness are afraid of. The session resulted in a great therapeutic breakthrough (Grof 2010, 288–93).

The exorcist Gabriele Amorth quotes a woman who is supposedly oppressed by the "evil spirit." What she thinks is a proof of the demon's influence seems to be rather a confirmation of the significance of her early childhood traumas: "I felt in me a mortal violence which was rooted in the distant past and which was repressed thanks to my upbringing. I held incomprehensible grudges, I wanted to scream, but I looked calm and sweet on the surface due to my habit of self-control. I had suicidal thoughts since adolescence, but they were always repressed. I lived in a state of constant anguish" (Amorth 2002, 92). Is not the idea of being possessed a defense mechanism that allows the individual to isolate himself from the painful awareness that the experienced traumas and the arising emotions are part of his own identity?

Exorcists emphasize that after an exorcism the person is generally composed and calm. In addition to all possible effects, exorcisms undoubtedly allow one to release the suppressed negative emotions. The existence of this purely therapeutic factor is also indicated by the fact that exorcisms often do not work immediately, but they must be repeated for many years, and even then the "liberation" may not be complete (Amorth 1997, 47). Amorth writes: "You get the impression that all the evil in the body must slowly come to light so that it can be completely removed" (Amorth 1997, 99).[5] The issue of "abreaction" of socially unaccepted feelings appears in psychiatry at least since the first therapies conducted by Breuer and Freud.

Because our culture is divided into the realm of religion and science, possession was addressed either from the perspective of materialistic neurology and psychiatry—usually stating that it is simply a "disease"—or from that of the doctrine of the Church, its anthropology and vision of the world. What did this mean? Both these institutions—science and the Church—are to some extent dogmatic. Neither of them can accept certain hypotheses or conclusions. For example, the Church cannot acknowledge that the devil that possesses may be a part of the human psyche, and science that the possessed person's psyche could be influenced in an external, extrasensory way. Therefore, one should look at possession from the third perspective. Possession must become a question about ourselves, a question that is: "Who is man, since he can be a possessed man?" And more psychologically: "How does our psyche really work, since it manifests such extraordinary processes as possession?"[6]

## Dissociation and Multiplicity

Are we unicity, or is our cohesion only an appearance? Many concepts and observations indicate that personality has aspects of multiplicity, not unicity.

The starting point of understanding possession is the fact that there are anti-thetical feelings, motives, subpersonalities or even the *alter ego* in the psyche. The tendencies opposite to the intended ones are visible in many ordinary life situations. Someone wants to pass his exam, and at the same time tends to fail it. He may feel deep in himself that he does not deserve it, that he has not learned enough, and that justice will be done only when he fails. He can be afraid of the failure, and at the same time need it. He is fully aware of the first of the opposite tendencies. The other may have a more complex structure, be unconscious, and arise on the basis of this part of the *ego*, which stands against individual intentions, meeting the requirements resulting from living in community, and which can be called conscience (Freud referred to it as the *superego*—it functions in each of us, and in more extreme cases manifests itself in the form of self-destructive tendencies). The weight and universality of countertendencies was also noted by Jung, who wrote:

> We can take this dichotomy of the human will, for which Bleuler has coined the term "ambitendency," as a constant factor, bearing in mind that the most primitive motor impulses are essentially antithetical, since, even in a simple act like stretching, the flexor muscles must be innervated. Normally, however, this ambitendency never leads to the inhibition or prevention of the intended act, but is absolutely necessary for its co-ordination and execution. (Jung 1976, 173)

So we are constantly divided. But are we divided to such a degree that we consist of separate subpersonalities? Or does dissociation occur only in pathological states? The concept of psychic dissociation or hidden personality appeared along with the theory and practice of animal magnetism promoted by Mesmer. His student, Armand-Marie-Jacques de Chastenet, Marquis de Puységur discovered that "magnetized" persons, in the state of "artificial somnambulism" (today we would say "hypnosis"), remembered the events that had occurred during the normal state, but in the normal state, they did not remember what they had done when in the trance. Puységur stated that it looked as if there had been two different existences in one person (Hart and Dorahy 2009, 4–5). The idea of psychic dissociation corresponds with the one of the unconscious (subconscious) and has functioned in psychology and psychiatry at least since the mid-nineteenth century (Whyte 1960; Dobroczyński 2001). In one of his earliest writings, in his 1893 article on hypnosis and hysterical symptoms, Freud wrote:

> How does a person with a healthy ideational life deal with antithetic ideas against an intention? With the powerful self-confidence of health, he suppresses and inhibits them so far as possible, and excludes them from his associations. This often succeeds to such an extent that the existence of an antithetic idea

against an intention is as a rule not manifest, but is only made probable when we come to consider the neuroses. [. . .] The antithetic idea establishes itself, so to speak, as a "counter-will," while the patient is aware with astonishment of having a will which is resolute but powerless. (Freud 1950, 38–40)

The ideas and impulses that are antithetical to the consciousness become suppressed, and the resistance of the *ego* makes them inaccessible. This is how—in short—the unconscious described by Freud is formed. A question arises: "What kind of life does the unconscious live?" Can something like the conscious *ego* shape itself under the threshold of consciousness? Freud opposes such a vision, yet even when he describes the *superego*, he personifies it very much. In his descriptions, the *superego* presses on the *ego*, demands from it, and, above all, observes it. A psychologist who emphasized the relative autonomy of the subconscious parts of the psyche was Pierre Janet, who claimed that in some states (hysteria, hypnotic trance, catalepsy) the personality splits and a subconscious personality—which becomes independent of the central personality—forms. Similarly, the author of the first intelligence test, Alfred Binet, believed that the fragments that form our personality can be disaggregated and gain their own consciousness, independent of the consciousness of the principal personality. Then the fragments can organize themselves into secondary personalities. Later, Ernest R. Hilgard, the author of the neo-dissociation theory (Hilgard 1977), dealt with the problem of divided consciousness. Using the conceptual apparatus of cognitive psychology, he postulates the existence of hierarchical ordering of "subordinate cognitive systems," each of which has relative unity and autonomy of function. These systems are directed by an overarching structure, that is, the *ego*. When for one reason or another—for example under the influence of hypnosis—the autonomy of the *ego* becomes constrained, one of the subordinate systems may take control of the individual's behavior.

In all of the approaches mentioned above, the basic model is similar. We deal with the division of psychic structures and contents, with the split elements being not merely repressed and unavailable to the consciousness. They do not remain amorphous, but group into aggregates and in some respects begin to resemble complete personalities. Jung attributed such quasi-personal aspects to complexes and archetypes. He wrote about archetypes:

They are spontaneous phenomena which are not subject to our will, and we are therefore justified in ascribing to them a certain autonomy. [. . .]. If that is considered, we are compelled to treat them as subjects; in other words, we have to admit that they possess spontaneity and purposiveness, or a kind of consciousness and free will. (Quoted in Tacey 2012, 255)

A psychic complex, according to Jung, is a group of unconscious emotions, fantasies, and motivational tendencies grouped around one or more archetypes characterized by a common emotional tone (Samuels, Shorter, and Plaut 1986, 34). For example, the father complex contains archetypal, universal content concerning the father figure and memory traces of relations with the father. Although a complex exists within our psyche, it is a semi-autonomous product and its activation may cause a very distinct change in human behavior.

A divided psyche was believed to play a part in mediumship, automatic writing, hypnosis, and "magnetic trance." A psychologist, naturalist, inventor, and popular hypnotherapist, Julian Ochorowicz, wrote about hypnotic somnambulism:[7]

> In somnambulism, there is always a change of character, and sometimes a completely new *ego* is formed, with which one must communicate separately. The somnambulist feels differently, so he thinks differently too. He speaks about his normal state as a second person, that he criticizes and very often condemns. [. . .] after awakening there is amnesia, i.e., he usually does not remember what he did when asleep. In the face of such easy oblivion, we would have the right to call somnambulant acts unwitting or non-conscious—but this is a matter of convention and there is no mistake if some authors refer to somnambulism as the *second state of consciousness*. What is also worth noting is the fact that amnesia does not usually work both sides: when he wakes up, the somnambulist (the hypnotized) does not remember what he did in his sleep, but in a sleep, he remembers what he did when he was awake. (Ochorowicz 1996, 84)[8]

Conversion symptoms, somnambulant and hypnotic states, and what is referred to today as dissociative identity disorder, if they were not associated with the influence of a spirit or demon, invariably connoted a peculiar vision of "becoming independent" of ourselves.[9] Nietzsche, like Feuerbach, saw the source of religion in the process of dissociation of mental states. He wrote:

> The psychological logic is this: when a man is suddenly and overwhelmingly suffused with the *feeling of power*—and this is what happens with all great affects—it raises in him a doubt about his own person: he does not dare to think himself the cause of this astonishing feeling—and so he posits a stronger person, a divinity, to account for it. [. . .] and like a sick man who, feeling one of his limbs uncommonly heavy, comes to the conclusion another man is lying on top of him, the naive *homo religiosus* divides himself into several persons. [. . .] religion is the product of a doubt concerning the unity of the person, an *altération* of the personality: in so far as everything great and strong in man has been conceived as superhuman and external, man has belittled himself—he has separated the two sides of himself, one very paltry and weak, one very strong

and astonishing, into two spheres, and called the former "man," the latter "God." (Nietzsche 1968, 86–87)

So religion would be born from the fact that a person feels internally divided; he considers certain spheres of himself to be alien and projects them into the images of gods. Also, Christian mystics, to describe their unusual experiences, often referred to the division of the soul (Dobroczyński 2001). St. Teresa of Avila says that:

> Though the soul is known to be undivided, it is fact and no fancy and often happens. Interior effects show for certain that there is a positive difference between the soul and the spirit, although they are one with each other. There is an extremely subtle distinction between them, so that sometimes they seem to act in a different manner from one another. (St. Teresa of Avila 1921, 268–69)

Psychoanalysts postulate that one person may have psychotic and non-psychotic levels of personality; the insane *ego* can occur alongside the normal personality. They introduce concepts such as the "internal saboteur" or "pathological organizations" that can easily be referred to as the *alter ego* (Grotstein 1999, 28–50). The term "pathological organizations" refers to a situation in which narcissistic, omnipotent, and "bad" parts of the *self* dominate the remaining part of the personality. This is a kind of tyranny, though it can provide a labile mental balance and protect the withdrawn, more sensitive part of the *self*.

Patients themselves sometimes use the metaphor of the "other person" inside them. This "other person" may forbid the anorexic to eat, claiming that the girl is too fat, although she rationally knows that she is emaciated. The "other one" pushes the person with obsessive-compulsive disorder to perform compulsive activities, or "tempts" someone else not to look around when crossing the road. The "other one" resists the progress in therapy, does not want development, expects the patient's defeat and punishment for him. In cases of psychosis or more severe personality disorders, the "other one" acquires a particularly expressive form, becoming audible.

Is our internal division always associated with some degree of pathology, with something problematic? Or maybe we should come to terms with the fact that—as Hilgard says—the unity of consciousness is an illusion? Much of the clinical and experimental data indicates that some kind and degree of division of our psyche always occurs. Depending on the situation, we behave differently and present different faces of our personality, not to mention the extreme situations in which we are able to amaze or disappoint ourselves. It seems that the social life forces us to have one, consistent *ego*. This results from the fact that we have to present to other people a coherent picture of ourselves so that they can construct a clear representation of us and locate it in a defined place in their internal map of the world and relationships. In reality, however, we are not as cohesive as we think. Rather, there are forces in us that actively help us to maintain relative cohesion, the feeling of unity of the *ego* and of being an indivisible whole.

## THE SEMI-OPEN PSYCHE—PARTICIPATION

Searching for the causes of possession in the psyche does not mean that we have to ignore or simplify the associated unusual phenomena. We are not obliged to adopt the simplest model of the psyche. First of all, the psyche does not have to be perceived as an isolated monad. Experiencing and perceiving the psyche as a "spherical" and isolated soul is the result of a specific psychological process, which I refer to as *coiling up*. It leads to an idealization of our *ego*, which begins to be regarded as the whole subject. However—as we have known for a long time—the psyche, containing unconscious processes, does not amount to the *ego*. The subject is fractured and nonlocal. When he wrote about the sources of religion, Feuerbach spoke of man:

> He feels the torment of his needs, yet satisfies them without knowing whether the impulse to do so comes from within or without, whether he is satisfying himself or some outside being. Man with his ego or consciousness stands at the brink of a bottomless abyss; that abyss is his own unconscious being, which seems alien to him. (Feuerbach 2017, 311)

However, is the "unconscious being" really our own? There are many indications that it is not so well separated from the outside and other people as our *ego*. I define this dissolving of the psyche in the environment as *participation*. The basic concept that investigates this theme is Jung's collective unconscious theory. The collective unconscious is created of patterns of typical reactions to universal life situations, such as birth, struggle, suffering, love, fear, sex, or death. These patterns are common to all people and cultures, so they must have arisen from some connectedness between all people. Probably it is not an ordinary connectedness within the transmission of culture, language, and tradition, as these patterns reside in the unconscious and are innate. It must be a more unusual penomenon.

Besides Jungian concepts, there are other relevant theories and observations which indicate that our psyche is not clearly "localized" or that human psyches penetrate one another. Such a concept is the Family Unconscious—a notion introduced by psychologist Edward Bruce Bynum as a result of his observations of the functioning of families and their members. Bynum noticed that family members share the content of dreams, emotions, attitudes, or behavioral patterns. The author writes:

> After full sessions with families where all were present, we would work with parts or subsystems of the family. Often in these situations with siblings or parents "family secrets" would emerge. When the timing was right for these secrets to come out to the whole family, somehow everyone seemed to already have a vague image of the other's secret, even though these had never been openly mentioned. Such secrets often included the oddest of acts and the most intimate of fantasies. There seemed to be a shared central image, not fully located in any one person, but with each member having his or her own perception of it. I assumed that there must have been some nonverbal communication going on. (Taub-Bynum 1984, 4)

Grof, in the course of his research into different states of consciousness, discovered that people are able to experience identification with mothers and children during childbirth, wounded soldiers, with whole groups of people, with animals, and the biological life of the planet. From our point of view, identifications with ancestors are particularly interesting, which—as Grof states—are specific, detailed, and sometimes take the form of participation in events from the life of ancestors and are associated with full identification, including knowledge of body posture and facial expression, as well as thought and emotional processes. In many cases, objective studies have confirmed the information obtained in this way (Grof 2000).

Family constellations of a German therapist Bert Hellinger reach similar areas. Hellinger states that a family is a community of fate in which the younger want to unconsciously follow and experience the fate of the older family members (Hellinger, Weber, and Beaumont 1998). This transgenerational approach shows that we can be unconsciously connected with a person we did not even know about, because it can be, for example, our grandmother's child that died prematurely and was forgotten. This kind of relationship, referred to as entanglement, has a great impact on our emotions, health, and relationships, and we may be completely unaware of these causes. During workshops, systemic constellations prove that we are able to "receive" information from strangers, and even—whatever it may mean—from the deceased. During the workshops, people who represent the father, mother, brother, or any other member of the client's family, living or dead, re-create the real relationships, emotions, and attitudes present in that family, without knowing the family or having any information about it. Such phenomena were observed earlier by Gregory Bateson, Virginia Satir, and Sharon Wegscheider-Cruse, to name a few (Satir 1983; Satir, Bandler, and Grinder 1976; Wegscheider-Cruse, Higby, Klontz, and Rainey 1995).

The connections between living organisms, between people, and generally within all matter are more and more fully confirmed by science. Physics is more and more "nonlocal," which means that individual physical systems cannot be isolated from the influences of the entire universe (Musser 2015). There are also many experiments that confirm that a person can influence another one, regardless of the distance (Laszlo 2007; McTaggart 2008; Kelly and Kelly 2010).

## THE CURSE OF RELATIVES

Many exorcists consider a curse put on the future possessed to be one of the reasons of possession. Amorth writes:

> The most common and difficult cases that I have encountered involved parents or grandparents who cursed their children or grandchildren. (Amorth 1997, 139)[10]

The psychological aspect of possession manifests itself clearly here. For how would someone's curse become the way to possession, if not through influencing the psyche of the accursed? After all, nobody assumes human power over Satan. Why would family members—mainly parents or grandparents—have this particularly intensified power to harm, if not through specific psychological mechanisms? Above, I wrote that within a multigenerational family unconscious influences are particularly strong and often shape our fate. In order to understand the impact a curse may have, we can start with the "curses" which affect psychotherapeutic patients.[11] Curses can have a different degree of intentionality. At one end, there are words, whose purpose was not to "curse," but to the patient's mind they are just like a curse that negatively shapes his life. At the other extreme, there are relatively rare cases in which the desire to bring about the worst sufferings is fully conscious. Between these extremes there is the whole spectrum of negative and aggressive messages from parents to children. "You're useless," "You can't make it yourself"—many people have heard similar words. The power of their influence is amazing—a person is convinced that his parents were wrong, believes that his life will be different, and yet he follows their curse. Perhaps he cannot oppose the script, because it would involve the feeling that he completely lost his parents, that he renounced them. So if they said he is a "loser," he becomes a life loser. In this way he shows them: "I am what you wanted me to be, don't reject me more." A woman who was cruelly treated in childhood decides that she will raise her children differently. Soon, she notices that she acts in the same way, she even begins to shout with the voice of her aggressive mother. This phenomenon shows how difficult it is to get rid of the destructive influence of a parent.

The fact that parents, in a sense, may want their children dead, would certainly take the first place in the ranking of taboos (Welldon 2010, 80). It is a complicated and ambiguous matter, but it requires at least a partial elucidation. What is not verbalized in everyday life is one of the universal themes on the mythological plane. Myths often address parents' animosity towards children and their attempts to dispose of them. A good example is *Enūma Eliš*, the Babylonian creation epic. It tells a story of the time when the two primeval forces, Apsu (the male fresh waters) and Tiamat (the female salt waters), created the first gods. Soon, however, these gods became a nuisance for their parents. Then Apsu said to Tiamat:

> Their way has become painful to me, By day I cannot rest, by night I cannot sleep; I will destroy [them] and put an end to their way, that silence be established, and then let us sleep! (Quoted in Heidel 1963, 19)

A similar situation is described in the Greek myth of Cronus, who for fear of dethronement devoured his own offspring (Graves 2017). And does not the biblical narrative of the expulsion from paradise tell about the parent's aggression towards his children? This account also shows God's fear that the creature may become equal to the creator, the fear for His own position. Similarly in the case of Jesus—it was his Father who sent him to die.

Hellinger discovered that on the unconscious level, the parent can expect the child to "die for him" (Hellinger, Weber, and Beaumont 1998). Children, in an unconscious way, want to take over the difficulties from older members of the family, particularly parents, such as depression, sense of guilt, anxiety, or illness. As if they said inwardly: "I for you." This happens without any activity on the part of the parent, but in some cases the parent may, also inwardly and unconsciously, say to the child: "Yes, you for me. Take this for me. Die for me." In this case, the child is burdened doubly. Based on the observations made while facilitating family constellations, the author states that atopic dermatitis may arise as a result of a specific "curse"—the former partner of the child's parent is angry because of the separation and wishes his future offspring ill (Hellinger and Nehrebecki 2012, 167–69).

The mother's (or grandmother's) curse may be more destructive than that of the father. The relationship between the mother and the child is unique, because, from the biological point of view, the child emerges from the mother's body, and is almost united with it in the fetal period (Fromm 1998, 406). There remains a psychological trace of this biological dependence that the mother can use in a destructive way. The child always wants the mother to legitimize its existence, and if she refuses to do it, saying, for example, that she considered terminating the pregnancy, it will be very difficult for the child to believe in its right to live. The mother for the child is like an Indian goddess Kali—she seems to be the one who, giving life, can also take it away.[12] Usually, we do not realize how archaic or demonic her emotions and fantasies can be. Her relationship with the child may be far from the usual relationship of two people, because the mother may treat the child as part of herself, perceive its attempts at independence as unjustified, and oppose them.

## CONSTRUCTING A DEMON

Can a demon really be what plagues the possessed person? Or is it the products of the psyche and disorder? As I mentioned above, in my opinion, "intermediate states" are possible here. A part of personality constituted in the form of a demon does not have to be composed only of biographical elements of the psyche, but can be associated with other people in time and space. If we take both dissociation and *participation* into account, we have the possibility to analyze the unique state of possession. The third mechanism is *coiling up*, that is formation and personification.

A demon is a conglomeration of experiences, traumas, drives, words, and events in the lives of other people, especially members of the family understood in the transgenerational sense. All this is subjected to the process of personification. It is also connected with the dominant religious culture, which is a forceful centuries-old source of meaning and influence, affecting the unconscious of both believers and atheists.

Who becomes possessed? Probably the people in whom unaccepted thoughts and impulses, psychological injuries, and unconscious influence of the family system are particularly strong and unstructured. They could have been abandoned or sexually abused and in their family there may be negative transgenerational factors in the form of murders, unfinished traumas, or mourning. Because these matters pertain to past generations, they are impossible to find in the biography of the possessed person, yet they affect his psyche. This interpretation is also supported by the fact that many exorcists see transgenerational factors as important causes of possession. Within the psyche of the possessed, the traumatic experiences and the identification with their ancestors' traumas live their own lives. At this point, the process of *coiling up*, consisting in building compact, self-regulating aggregates, enters the stage. The impulses are personified, and become the building blocks of an alien personality, a "demon." This may take the form of dissociative identity disorder or possession.

It seems that the repressed contents and emotions have a natural tendency to accumulate and form quasi-personal complexes. This tendency may result from the human need to experience important things in an interpersonal relationship. Thanks to personification, dialogue becomes possible. Ochorowicz indicates an important element of the process of personification of the complex, which is giving a name to the dissociated part of the psyche. During hypnosis, it can consolidate suppressed drives and split content into a new "personality" (Ochorowicz 1996, 204). Jung identically presents this matter in his doctoral thesis. He writes that the question addressed to the medium ("Who says that?") is a suggestion that causes the synthesis of the subconscious personality (Jung 1991, 80). This context allows us to understand the old practice of asking about the demon's name. It had to be revealed during the exorcism (Amorth 1997, 100).

The demon, though terrifying, is much safer than being overwhelmed by an unstructured affect and the intergenerational sense of trauma. The devil is a blasphemer and a pervert, but as such he is known and, contrary to appearances, culturally accepted. There are ways of coping with him, such as exorcisms, and there are also people who are not afraid of him and understand his nature, i.e., exorcists. The demon-exorcism system allows the integration of absolutely antisocial, destructive impulses into the framework of society.

## PSEUDO-POSSESSION—CLINICAL CASE STUDY

Monica was twenty-six years old. She was diagnosed with paranoid schizophrenia, but she herself claimed to be possessed. She said that there were "Antichrist" and "Lucifer" in her. Antichrist was male, wanted to be skinny, and forbade her to eat. Her internal organs, skeleton, and "what is red" were built from him. Lucifer was female and encouraged her to eat. Lucifer created what is "white" in the body, i.e., adipose tissue, and was in "every cell." Lucifer and Antichrist hated each other.

Monica also claimed that she had to maintain her body weight between thirty-five and thirty-seven kilograms. When she started to put on weight, when her cheeks "became round," she had to slap herself. Eating was one of the main issues Monica concentrated on. She had had anorectic and bulimic episodes before (she had weighed as much as 80 kg), and for this reason she had to leave the convent she was in. She said she never "fully" ate, but only took food to her mouth, bit it, and then spit it out. Because she found it disgusting, she did it out of sight. She ate only those remnants she could not spit out. When she ate before going to sleep, she had—as she claimed—

nightmares (she remembered that in one of these dreams she had dreamed about a sausage, in another—about a drip and buns; when asked about her associations with these elements of the dream content, she replied: "debauchery, penises" in relation to the first dream, and "water" and "three fat women crushing me" as a reference to the other two elements). However, when she denied herself eating and maintained weight, she had "peaceful and blissful dreams" in which she saw "heaven."

Monica claimed she was not human because her body was built from Antichrist and Lucifer. She said she was "part-woman, part-man," which was internally consistent, given that Lucifer and Antichrist were of different sexes. She said that Lucifer "is a condom on Antichrist" and "a condom must be thin." She claimed she was built from an inverted cross, surrounded by rosary beads. She was also the unity of the "body," "psyche" and "soul," and could "talk on three levels," that is, on the "divine" and "human" level, and the one of Antichrist and Lucifer. She said that "all hell" was located in her, but "God allowed it." And when the world ends, there will be "heaven" in her and on earth.

Monica initially refused to take medicines, she claimed that she was all "chemistry" after the medicines she had taken before. These drugs, according to her, caused holes in her stomach, and made her vomit.[13] She decided to go to the hospital, but she claimed that her illness was a "spiritual illness," not a mental one. That is why she wanted to be treated "unconventionally," through hypnosis.

During one of the therapeutic sessions, Monica "turned into" Antichrist. She began to speak with a hoarse voice, tilted her head, twisted her face. She swore at me and said: "You want to destroy me." After this rather short episode, she was aware of what had happened—when I asked her, "who it was a moment ago," she replied: "Antichrist."

When the neuroleptics administered to her slowly eliminated psychotic symptoms (which does not mean that they cured her psyche), Monica's psychopathology became more and more similar to the image of anorexia. Monica no longer explained that her reluctance to eat was because of the influence of "Antichrist," but there appeared rationalizations typical of anorexia, such as reluctance to put on weight. So it looks like the mechanisms of anorexia were used by psychosis. Psychosis modified the conflicts experienced by Monica in such a way that her unconscious tendencies and motives became personified and mythologized.

What the anorexic experiences in the form of conflicting tendencies, Monica felt as the conflict of two mythological personalities. Every anorexic—as I demonstrated in the chapter on anorexia—is in a sense "part-woman, part-man." She cannot fully accept the female identity and assumes some archetypically masculine traits. Also, the anorexic experiences a conflict between two contradictory tendencies, almost two different "persons." One of my patients during mental work referring to her body, had the impression that her body was equally divided into two parts: the right side felt healthier, nourished and located as if above, the left—as the reverse of the right side—a "withered branch." She also said she had the impression that she nourished only one side of the stomach while the other was hungry.

Monica once said, still in the psychotic phase of the disease, that Antichrist "affected" her "through her mother and sister" and that then she began to tremble. Here, one can detect a conflict with her mother (as well as with her sister, as a woman, a person associated with the mother, and perhaps for other reasons too), also described in the chapter on anorexia. Antichrist that appears within this relationship is male and forbids eating. Is this not a symbolic expression of the negation of femininity?

Monica's delusions were not based solely on general religious awareness; she had never encountered similar considerations in her life. Probably the collective, archetypal level of her unconscious contributed to the creation of these visions. The content presented by Monica focused on two areas: religion and sex. The symbolism of her delusions referred to sexual intercourse. Lucifer, being female, was a condom on Antichrist. So it was an obvious symbol of sexual intercourse. Imagine now an inverted cross surrounded by rosary beads. This image can have the same meaning. The masculine element and feminine one, Antichrist and Lucifer, were in conflict. This was also Monica's internal conflict. Perhaps she saw it could be stopped through a sexual act. However, she reached a substitute of this act of synthesis and temporary calmness when she maintained her weight within certain limits.

## POSSESSION—CLINICAL CASE STUDY

Sylvia was admitted to hospital after an attack of uncontrollable rage, during which she destroyed objects in the apartment and threatened the people in her vicinity. According to the witnesses of this incident, she shouted out curses in a changed, low voice, at the same time threatening to kill them and to jump out the window. When I met her in the psychiatric ward, she was twenty-eight years old, and she was considered possessed by the Church for over a year. The first episode of illness occurred one and a half years before our first conversation. The episode took place during a special mass in one of the churches, where people prayed for "cleansing the body and soul." Sylvia got a seizure then. She did not remember the incident afterwards; she heard about it from the witnesses. Soon after, regular prayers for her liberation and then exorcisms began. During these activities Sylvia went into a trance, raged and, with foam on her lips, destroyed religious symbols (as she claimed, only those that were blessed). By all accounts, she had so much physical strength then that even a few men could not stop her. She would also go into a trance when there were prayers in her absence, but for her intention.

According to the priest who exorcised Sylvia, she displayed supernormal knowledge, talking about the "sins" of the people she did not know (he stated that her claims were true in his case). He also said about Sylvia's reaction to the cross of Saint Benedict that he carried with him. At the time of the exorcism, Satan reportedly said through her mouth, "I gave him poison." At first, the priest did not know what these words could mean, but later he read that when one day St. Benedict had blessed the food before the meal, his cup had broken. As it turned out, there had been poison in it.

During exorcisms, Sylvia reportedly spoke Latin and Hebrew. She also talked about her extraordinary abilities. She said she could levitate, walk on a vertical wall, had photographic memory, and could remotely influence people. One of the doctors claimed that she had put an elderly, restless patient to sleep; and that she had done it in an instant, bringing her hands close to that patient's head. Making a gesture with her hand, she also made the same patient walking down the corridor—a few meters away from her—turn back and go to her room.

I had the opportunity to observe one of Sylvia's attacks. It was shortly after two visiting priests had left her room. Sylvia was sitting on the bed, leaning against the wall and rhythmically hitting it with the back of her head. She was trembling. When a nurse and I laid her down, she had her eyes closed and was wriggling in all directions, also taking positions similar to the hysterical arch.[14] She began to thrash and struggle more and more. Her eyes were rolled back. Finally, in a low voice, she began to unintelligibly mumble, and a bit of foamy saliva appeared on her lips. The first phase of the attack ceased. She lay quiet now, but did not react in any way to the words spoken to her. The second phase of the attack began. Sylvia, all shivering and with foam on her lips, said in a low, "satanic" voice: "Go away, this whore is mine." I asked, "Who is supposed to go away?" "The priest," she replied. When after a while she repeated the order, I asked her, "'Mine'? Whose exactly?" After this question Sylvia froze for a moment, then slowly began, totally contorted, sitting up. When she reached the semi-sitting position, her head was unnaturally twisted. She looked at me with the whites of her eyes, and the expression on her face said only one thing to me, "What is it, don't you know?" As if she had unmasked my insincerity and the fact that I did not want to take an answer seriously. The entire attack took about five minutes. She came around, forgetting everything. During another attack, when the physician addressed her by her name, she responded in a changed voice, "She's not here."

Sylvia defined her childhood as "good," but she could not recall any details.[15] She was brought up mainly by her mother and grandmother, because her father was often absent and later moved out. She could not say much about her relations. She only said that the relationship with her mother was "good." When her father tried to make contact with her recently, she told him that she did not expect it, that she was "indifferent" to him. Sylvia as a fourteen-year-old got to a local sect and remained involved in it continuously for ten years. The decision to join the sect was influenced by the desire for a deeper relationship with a fatherly man, which she admitted herself. She was fascinated by the guru's personality and, as she called them, "tricks." She also learned various kinds of parapsychic techniques, such as telepathy or precognition. However, after some time, as she said, she felt that "all these were just tricks," that she wanted something different, a contact with a "higher being." She left the sect and hid in a Catholic convent for one year. However, the Catholic religion did not suit her "completely." So she joined the Hare Krishna movement and stayed in that community for several years. Being in this religious movement, she began studying at a Jesuit high school. She wanted to learn "the ways of reaching Christians" there.

One day, someone persuaded her to take part in a pilgrimage. The group of pilgrims was informed that among them there was a person who hesitated about faith. They prayed that Sylvia would fully accept the Catholic faith. As the pilgrims approached the sanctuary, Sylvia felt that the necklace she wore (from Hare Krishnas) closed more and more around her neck. She asked some people to unclasp it, but because it was impossible, they had to cut it. She remembered that she was crying at the time, but she could not say anything about the emotions that accompanied that situation. The pilgrimage took place two years before Sylvia's hospitalization, and between these events she worked for some time in a parish office.

Sylvia did not take a clear position on what was happening to her. Her behavior and statements indicated an ambiguous attitude to the question of "possession"; she doubted in the demonological theory presented to her by the Church. Here is what she said, for example, about "possession": "Somehow it's difficult for me to accept it, these are like things from a horror movie." On the other hand, I saw that Sylvia, in some subtle way, took relish in her "possession."

Similarly, she had contradictory attitudes towards the Church—despite the negation of its teaching, she maintained the contact with it (see Amorth 2002, 154 et seq.). When she spoke about the Host, there was a tone of nonchalance in her voice. For example, she said: "Well, this wafer, I don't know what they call it" (she could only say the word "wafer," but not "Host"). At the same time, she claimed, there was something like an ironic laughter in her. When asked to name her emotions in relation to the Host, she was only able to say "shit," "disgusting." As if she were not allowed to think about this object. Everything she could express was contained in the word "shit." She claimed that nothing else came to her mind. On the other hand, she showed a dogmatic belief in the supernatural nature of the Host when she said: "Substantially it's just flour and water, but I mean what's behind it." However, when I asked her what was behind it, she could not answer. Also, she could not say the word "God," or "Jesus," who she referred to as a "puppet on a tree" (meaning the crucifix). When she opened the Bible, she saw—as she said—only white, empty pages.

Generalized "ambivalence" was noticeable in her entire way of being (in the content she communicated, in its emotional expression, in the functioning in the therapeutic relation). It manifested psychological dissociation, some of which could be noticed even when Sylvia behaved "normally," that is, between her attacks. For instance, when in the first session she told me her story, her face took on a characteristic expression that any attentive observer would associate with a feeling of grief or pain. However, when asked what she felt, she replied that she did not feel anything. This is of course nothing unusual, this type of cutting off from emotions is very common. However, it should be noted that in the case of Sylvia, "dissociative elements" were permanent. She remembered how, after leaving the sect, "her legs carried her" to the Hare Krishna temple. She claimed she had tried to change the direction or stop, but she failed. There was also an opposite situation—she could not take a step to approach the Catholic confessional.

Sylvia's pseudoparalysis before confession is a typical example of conversion movement disorder. Certainly, the first of the described phenomena, i.e., automatic, impossible to stop, walking, is much rarer. Paralysis is the involuntary reaction of a group of muscles that we can treat as related to unconscious reluctance or fear of confession. This reaction is rather simple, but if we take into account the fact that there is a hidden intention behind it, we can consider it to be a manifestation of dissociation. Automatic walking would be a more complex behavior associated with both motoric behavior and cognitive activity. Perhaps in this case we deal with greater autonomy of the dissociated part of the personality, which would mean that the mental complex has been "personified" to a greater degree.

When the exorcisms began, Sylvia initially still suffered from various conversions (she could not walk, she lost her voice), then these phenomena ceased and the attacks of possession started. It seems that the unconscious tendencies were split off to a larger degree, and were no longer manifested by isolated symptoms, but in the form of a personified complex, "Satan." A symptomatic continuum can be observed here, from generalized seizures (first attack), through conversions, to full-blown possession.

Sylvia had another attack during her hospitalization. She attacked the priest who came with the sacrament of Eucharist. She cursed him and struggled with him. However, she did not show "superhuman" strength this time. Also, after the attack ceased, she partly remembered it (perhaps this unusual change was caused by anticonvulsants. It is also possible that psychotherapy and the atmosphere of the ward played a role here too). Although she did not remember what she had said, Sylvia kept the visual memories of this event. She also remembered her aggression. I believe that what happened to her during that attack was a manifestation of a smaller degree of dissociation of her psyche. The "Satan" complex was partly depersonalized, which means that Sylvia integrated some of the psychological elements that had built it into her basic *self*. As a "more complete" person, she kept the memory and confronted her aggression.

Amorth makes a distinction between "possession" and "demonic oppression" in the way that he includes people who after an exorcism (so after an attack) do not remember what happened to them in the first category, and those who have vague memories of this state in the other one (Amorth 1997, 84). If we followed the above distinction in the case of Sylvia, we would have to conclude that pharmacotherapy or a different psychological situation changed the demonic influence. Of course, this would be inconsistent with the theological claims.

During her stay in the convent, in the periods when nuns prepared for masses and other religious activities, Sylvia had an impression that the atmosphere around her became "heavy" ("as if I were to go through cotton wool"). Then she was suddenly in the mood to laugh. The impressions of a "heavy atmosphere," "going through cotton wool" and the fact that, in reaction to them, Sylvia wanted to laugh, seem to be meaningful. We have the feeling of such a "heavy" atmosphere when we assume that our spontaneity will be rejected and stigmatized. How does it relate to Sylvia's experiencing? Religious symbols meant repression for her. We are not able to retrace this repression, but it seems that it is about sexuality in this case. Sylvia, as we know, joined the sect at the age of fourteen, at puberty, when the sex drive invariably comes into play. She said that she had begun to feel it clearly then. It could not be satisfied, however. Moreover, Sylvia did not even have the opportunity to theoretically familiarize herself with issues related to sex. Instead, she was ordered to suppress sexual impulses with meditation and mantras (when I talked to her, she claimed that she was still a virgin). Sexual needs, although suppressed, could not disappear, they rather formed a hidden current in her psyche. In the convent, there was also no room for expressing her "other side." Perhaps within the "Satan" complex, in a camouflaged form, Sylvia satisfied her dissociated drives. His figure, by his very nature, is a negation of the repressive components of religion.

Sylvia once said that a "voice" said something to her when she was looking at the crucifix hanging in the ward library. She quoted to me: "That fucker was not a man." This hallucination can also be a sign of the repressed sexual impulses. After all, the "voice" blamed Jesus for "not being a man," meaning he did not represent the sexual aspect. Sylvia attacked religion, inter alia, for not allowing to fulfill sexual desires. Another event can also be indicative of Sylvia's repressed sexual needs. Once a friend of hers, supposedly a Satanist, reportedly offered her ritual intercourse on Good Friday, after which they were to commit suicide together. Sylvia did not agree. She admitted, however, that she was sexually attracted to that man. On Good Friday she had a great attack (she was in another psychiatric ward then). It is difficult to say if her attack was caused by the recurrence of the suppressed drive or by the symbolic weight of the holiday itself. Maybe both of these factors played a role here.

Through all of our meetings, Sylvia did not show unambiguous emotions. I could just observe signs of suppressed or overt aggression, but only during the attack. The first time she manifested her emotions was in a joint session with her mother. The mother was a simple Catholic woman who accepted the demonological concept of possession without reservation. It was obvious that she suffered a lot because of what was happening to her daughter. During our meeting, she asked anxiously whether Sylvia was still in contact with the people from the sect, she asked her to renounce Satan. What did I observe during this session? First of all, it struck me that Sylvia stopped being "demonic," which she had emanated before, and which—probably partly consciously—she tried to maintain. She sat as if "huddled up" inside, isolated from her mother, not answering her questions and not responding to her attempts to talk. There was a great distance between the mother and the daughter, also on the intellectual level. The mother's confidence that her daughter was possessed by the devil seemed to increase this distance. The theory that Sylvia had previously been willing to recognize now became an obstacle to their communication. I had the impression that Sylvia felt deep sadness and resentment, realizing that the mother also could see her and her problems only through the prism of possession. Noticing this, I intervened, asking Sylvia if she felt the need to be understood. "I think everyone feels it," she replied and began to cry. Her behavior had never seemed so natural before.

Sylvia showed some hysterical personality traits (*ICD-10*, 173).[16] People with this personality disorder have a tendency of dramatization, shallowness and lability of mood, vulnerability to suggestions, constant search for new incentives, a disposition to fantasize, and egocentrism. In such patients, various forms of "dissociation" can be observed (formerly hysteria was closely related to dissociative conversion disorders, and although now these states are not equated with each other, the original approach was not without foundation). This often manifests itself as a kind of sexualization of the contact without directly addressing sexual issues at the same time. The patient introduces implicit, but easily identifiable sexual content, and on the other hand, she "does not admit" it. And if the therapist pointed to this aspect of her behavior, she would reject the interpretation with indignation.[17]

Sylvia often said she wanted to "get rid of these things," that is, her paranormal abilities, and that she wanted to be "normal." On the other hand, one could sense an element of bragging about these skills. She reported the unusual phenomena that happened to her (undoubtedly realizing that she impressed the listener), and at the same time showed inadequate nonchalance and a kind of "lack of interest" in the affairs she was talking about.[18] She acted as if none of these things really concerned her. This behavior was like that of hysterical women, with the difference that instead of talking about superhuman powers, they introduce the sexual aspect. Sylvia, like those patients, constantly used her words and behaviors to emphasize the element from which she also permanently isolated herself, pretending to be "naive."

The behavior described above can also be seen as a manifestation of the defense mechanism used by Sylvia, namely projective identification (see Hinshelwood 1991, 179 et seq.). By projecting elements of her emotional life onto another person, Sylvia wanted to take control of him. So she aroused interest in someone with her "paranormality," and then "disavowed" the fact that she was talking about something unusual. In this way, her own emotions, for example fascination, were experienced by another person. In such a situation she gained control over that person, because she controlled his mental state and had the impression of better control over her own psyche. This basic mechanism is well known: for instance, we often calm down when someone else gets angry. As if he took the anger from us. Sylvia had a tendency to search her own qualities in another person, and getting the impression that she "knew" that person, she thought that she could manipulate him.[19] In her opinion, one of the doctors "looked down" on the patients and was "messed up." When she saw "anti-ecclesiasticism" in her, she experienced a strong desire to "somehow enter her" and "harm her internally."

Sylvia was overwhelmed by the desire to control and dominate. She tried to practice magic, she wrote pacts with the devil in which she surrendered to him in order to obtain his power. She said that she had once made a wax figure that symbolized a friend of hers, and then punctured it and cut its legs off; she reportedly met that man two months later—in a wheelchair, without legs. Some time after Sylvia left the hospital, I heard that she, in her stories, had portrayed me as a psychologist who, under her hypnotic influence, walked on his hands. These stories (I do not know to what extent she believed in them) show the strength of her need to manipulate.

## NOTES

1. See Mt 8:28–34; Mk 5:1–20; Lk 8:26–39; Mt 9:32–34; Mt 17:14–21; Mk 9:14–29; Lk 9:37–42.

2. Quotation translated from Polish by Barbara Gąstoł.

3. However, Christians recognize the possibility of acting under inspiration.

4. *The Exorcist* ["Egzorcysta"] monthly released in Poland publishes interviews with exorcists, testimonies of the freed persons, historical and ecclesiastical articles, biblical exegeses. Each issue addresses a phenomenon that may purportedly lead to possession, such as bioenergetic therapy, occultism, astrology, and heavy metal music, as well as hypnosis or Bert Hellinger's systemic constellations.

5. Quotation translated from Polish by Barbara Gąstoł.

6. Also, if we analyze the cases of murders, perversions, bizarre bestiality, which after all are not so rare, we can build a slightly different picture of man. As we know from history, quite ordinary people were capable of unimaginable bestiality (an example can be the Volhynia slaughter dated 1943–1945, during which entire families were murdered with saws, axes, scythes, and hammers).

7. The term "somnambulism" means sleepwalking, but is also used to describe the deep phase of hypnosis (see Kratochvíl 1996, 53–55).

8. Quotation translated from Polish by Barbara Gąstoł.

9. There are many disorders with dissociative symptoms known to psychiatry (see Jakubik 1979, 302–15; Wciórka 2002b, 429–30). For instance, Ganser syndrome, observed in soldiers, prisoners, and other people in difficult situations, is characterized by giving wrong—though close to correct—answers, doing things incorrectly, and partial amnesia for recent events (these people may specifically "protest" against the frustrating, restrictive situation they are in). Other disorders of the dissociative nature include: puerilism—the behavior that mimics that of a small child; dissociation fugue—amnesia for one's identity accompanied by an unexpected action; somnambulism; and even—in my opinion—bedwetting in children, which is a manifestation of regression. The bedwetting children I worked with were in some respects "too mature." Perhaps their nocturnal incontinence was to balance that untimely, burdening "maturity" (at night they became "infants"). A high percentage (30%) of somnambulists among such children is characteristic (Jakubik 1979, 310–11), which perhaps confirms the existence of "another life" in them. Of course, the most spectacular manifestation of dissociation is the dissociative identity disorder, the so-called mul-

tiple personality (Fauman 1994, 271–72). In this case, there are temporary changes in personality causing that the person literally becomes "someone else." In each of the possible states, he has different memories, lifestyle, interests, other abilities.

10. Quotation translated from Polish by Barbara Gąstoł.

11. One can also point to ritual curses of the kind described by Marcel Mauss under the name "the idea of death suggested by the collectivity." Mauss describes the cases of death when someone violated a taboo or was bedeviled. In such cases, the person believes he must die and actually dies. The author claims that such a person loses contact with the sacred powers and things that normally sustained him (Mauss 2001, 337–57). Perhaps some psychological mechanisms are similar in the case of ritual and family curses, after all both types concern "protective powers."

12. Probably a mother tends to be more threatening to a girl. Freud notes that women's fear of being killed or devoured by the mother is regularly reported in the course of analysis. Freud explains this as a projection of the girl's aggression towards her mother, but also mentions the possibility that the daughter perceives her mother's unconscious hostility (Freud 1997c, 186, 196).

13. Actually, these statements do not have to be far from the truth—whoever sees how neuroleptics generally work, he must admit that these metaphors are close to reality.

14. The hysterical arch (*arc de cercle*)—a characteristic position of the body taken during attacks of hysteria, characterized by the body bent backwards and the tension of many muscle groups. Wilhelm Reich considered the hysterical arch to be a somatic symptom of suppressed sexuality, because the body response associated with orgasm is the opposite (Reich 1961, 306–307).

15. Such a general statement, with the inability to remember details (regarding specific moments of early relationships with caretakers), usually indicates a deep dysfunction of the child's bond with its relatives.

16. *ICD-10* does not do this, but many psychoanalytic studies distinguish between hysterical and histrionic personality disorder (see Gabbard 2000, 557–61), considering the latter to be the deeper one (more primary defense mechanisms such as splitting and projective identification, as well as weaker social adaptation, worse intellectual and life functioning of the histrionic patients). In this case, I am not able to make such a distinction (there are both histrionic and hysterical features here).

17. Hysteria was called *"la grande simulatrice,"* i.e., the great imitator; the name resulted from the fact that the symptoms of hysteria imitate many symptoms of somatic diseases. Vagueness and "fakery" builds this disorder also on the psychological level. This immanent "fake" can be noticed on many levels, from the above-mentioned masking through the conversion symptoms of somatic disorders, the artificiality of the demonstrative expression of emotions, to the simple tendency to deviate from the truth. A closer look at some conversions also reveals ambiguity: they may be something on the verge of involuntary reaction and intentional simulation. An example can be conversion seizures, which resemble epilepsy, but usually there is no tongue biting, involuntary urination, or wounding during the fall. So although it is certainly not consciously controlled behavior, it seems that there is a certain level of volitional interference in it. Another example is the moment of convulsions or faint-

ing. Here again, although we do not deal with pure manipulation, the attitude of the people around and the benefits that can be obtained from such a demonstration have a significant impact that triggers the symptom.

18. Which corresponds to the famous *la belle indifference* (a term coined by Janet) of hysterical patients, that is, relative indifference even towards their symptoms that cause significant disability.

19. This squares with the observation of the exorcist, who states that the persons under the demon's power "feel that they can influence others' lives, wishing them ill with a meanness, almost a dominance, that comes from within" (Amorth 1997, 40).

*Chapter Seven*

# Spirits, Soul, Immortality

## SPIRITS OF THE DEAD AND
## A PATHOLOGICAL CULT OF ANCESTORS

### Spirits—Entities and Projections

In this book, I do not intend to investigate the issue of possible existence of "spiritual entities," let alone the issue of "life after death," but I would like to shed some light on these cases of manifestation of the "deceased" in which the psychological mechanism of the whole phenomenon can be identified. From the psychopathological point of view, the "spirits" discussed in this chapter take two basic forms. The first one is simply the hallucinations of spirits. The other one includes more diverse, psychological phenomena, where the impact of the deceased person on the patient manifests itself. This impact goes beyond the mere memories or experiences associated with mourning. Often, it may be an involuntary imitation of the deceased person (usually the parent) or a feeling of being prepossessed by him to varying degrees. It turns out that the internal image of the late person can have an extremely strong, sometimes destructive impact. I observe this phenomenon in people whose parent died, and their previous relations with the parent were not good. The parent hurt them, rejected them, or deprived them of their independence. But in this way, paradoxically, he indelibly tied them to himself.

The issue of the continued existence and functioning of the dead in our world, that is the issue of "spirits of the dead," occurs in most religions. In the religions of primitive cultures—where the basic objects of worship were various "spirits" (spirits of totemic ancestors, nurturing and harmful spirits)—great importance was attached to preventing the negative impact of the dead on the living. Reading the writings of anthropologists leads to the conclusion that the matter of eliminating the deceased's soul from the world, or at least neutralizing its negative aspects, is an important motive of funeral rituals. The natives say it outright, but even when they define their motivation as an attempt to ensure that the deceased have a happy journey to the afterlife (Szyjewski 2000, 195, 199), one can assume the same causes, at least as coexisting. It may even be that the bodies of the people whose spirits are considered powerless and unable to harm are not buried at all and are left at the place of death (Szyjewski 2000, 198). In most cases, however, traditional peoples use complex rites.

Funeral rituals can be treated as equivalents of initiation (Szyjewski 2000, 196), helping an individual to cut off from his current status, the status of a living person in this case. Their goal is to force the spirit to separate itself from the past life and leave the world of the living. For this purpose, mourners dance, shout, cry, describe the charms of the land of the dead, and encourage the spirit to leave. Szyjewski writes:

> The ceremonial frame of the ritual incorporates grief and the desire to have the deceased stay, and at the same time the instinctive aversion consisting in trying to recede and purify oneself as soon as possible. (Szyjewski 2000, 196)[1]

Looking at the issue from the psychological perspective, it is not the spirit that is a threat to the community and it does not want to defend against it, it is the unconscious mental processes of its members that are the threat. Rituals are aimed at indirect expression of unconscious desires and emotions as well as their structuring and closure.

Freud explained that the phenomenon of the belief in spirits of the deceased resulted from the projection of hidden hostility, which after the death of a loved one is experienced particularly painfully (Freud 2004). He indicated that every relationship, even the most loving one, contains an element of hostility, even a wish for the death of the beloved person. When death really comes, there is a huge sense of guilt and the projection (that is perceiving hostility as occurring on the part of the deceased) protects from it. This mechanism creates a "spirit," because the persistence of aggression and sense of guilt causes continuous re-creation of the illusion that the late person exists. Of course, the greatest intensity of difficult emotions towards relatives can be expected in people with mental—e.g., neurotic—problems (anger due to prolonged dependence, traumas, lack of sufficient love, etc.).

The psychological background that conditions the cultural belief in spirits may be similar to that which leads to "psychopathological" contact with the dead. So primitive peoples can be motivated to celebrate their rites by the fear of what actually happens to neurotics.

## Hallucination and the Relationship

Psychiatrists usually treat hallucinations as phenomena of only negative consequences for patients, because the latter often complain that these symptoms are awkward. Thus, they do not notice that hallucinations—being projections of the psychic elements of the patient—must also fulfill some positive functions within the psyche.[2] Hallucinations are not accidental products, and the fact that they take similar forms in various people proves that they are based on universal psychic structures. These structures do not manifest themselves during normal life; only the disorder allows their identification. A hallucination can have a homeostatic aspect even when it noticeably disturbs some area and is perceived as something unpleasant by the subject. Emphasizing the negative effect of hallucinations, the psychiatrist says, for example, that "the patient attempted to commit suicide because he was forced by the imperative voices he heard."[3] However, understanding the issue this way, he actually follows the psychotic reasoning—he adopts the "person–external voice" pattern of thinking. And yet the individual is not "isolated" from the "voice" he hears, but in one way or another it is his voice. Even if the "voice" disappears, it does not mean that the patient will stop having suicidal tendencies. If it disappears, they can even intensify, because the problems will stop being projected outside the subject.

A hallucination can serve as a substitute for a relationship with another person. For some patients, the hallucinated figures remain the closest "people" to them. It does not even matter here that these hallucinations can be nagging, and that the appearing figures are aggressively or critically oriented toward the hallucinating person. Sometimes, because of the patient's previous experiences, they cannot be different. It is another example of the principle that the existence of a relationship is more important than its quality. The psyche is formed and functions within interpersonal relationships, and this relationality remains important forever. Probably we all happened to say something to ourselves, as if thinking was not enough. Lonely people often talk to themselves and even conduct imaginary conversations. They need this exteriorization of thoughts to be able to function. If the whole of their internal situation did not change, and they were only "cured" from this form of dealing with loneliness, then they would really go insane.

The same concerns those who experience auditory or visual hallucinations. These products contain part of their lives, they are personified memories, past experiences, and relationships with important persons. Sometimes they consist of a memory of one person, sometimes they are an "eclectic" product, built of different people and events. Sometimes the patient says that he wants to see the figure and does not want to get rid of his hallucinations. A twenty-year-old girl, who developed a deep personality disorder on the basis of traumatic situations of early childhood, hallucinated strange figures that she then drew. Her drawings showed faces that looked like a hybrid of a newborn and a stereotypical depiction of an alien (they had a large skull, a small jaw, protruding cheekbones, large eyes). The patient wanted to believe that what she saw was her "guardian angel." When we worked on her associations with those drawings, she thought of her grandmother, who had looked after her until she was five. She was the only person who showed her real warmth. She said she wanted the hallucinated faces to talk to her like "people," not just speak in broken sentences or single words. At that stage, she did not want her hallucinations to disappear. They had a great advantage over people, which she emphasized herself—they could always be with her. One can see the stabilizing function of hallucinations here.

What we generally call a hallucination forms a continuum. It consists of fantasies, vague impressions, weak "inner voice," voices "in the head" (so-called pseudohallucinations), and hallucinations in the strict sense. Often the strength of the hallucination—its location on the above continuum—depends on the attitude of the one who listens to the patient. The psychiatrist's standard vocabulary includes the question: "Do you hear voices?" This approach does not allow for a nuanced observation—the patient can either hide his sensations or is forced to utter them in an extremely unambiguous form.

The aforementioned girl fantasized that her father was Hannibal Lecter, the demonic character of *The Silence of the Lambs*. The fantasy gave her a special satisfaction. However, she did not just fantasize—she felt his presence, periodically heard him talking to her, hallucinated his figure. She claimed, for example, that he was talking to her when she was on the bus, but no one else saw or heard him. There were many similar statements suggesting that she "saw" Lecter during her psychotherapy. The patient said, for example, that he was in the office during the session, described his facial expressions, movements. However, during one of the meetings, when I suggested that she saw Lecter, she was surprised. "No, I've never seen him. I know he exists, but I didn't see him." How to interpret this?

Our insight into hallucinations as quite similar to normal visual perception is simplified. It is very difficult to determine how much the patient really "sees" a given figure. Often there seems to be a kind of "irresistible sense of presence" that is probably primary in relation to the visual image. The fact that the patient talks about the image may be more a product of that sense and linguistic habit than real visual experiences. It is our language limitation that can cause that the only way to express the experience is to say we "see" something.

Now, to return to our patient. Although Lecter was only brutal towards her, she felt his protection as well. This points to the complex issue of benefits that can be derived from a traumatic relationship, and in this case additionally imaginary. The patient had a brutal, unpredictable, and probably psychotic father, who eventually disowned her. The relationship with him became the cornerstone of her problems. Suppressed anger, resentment, and unfulfilled need for care still existed in her psyche in relation to his figure. She could not count on someone other than Lecter to help, because only he was like her father. Any other person would be an unrealistic fantasy, no one else would contain her projected aggression. When she received therapeutic help from me, she did not know how to deal with it. Sometimes she tried to see me as sadistic and cold, then she smiled, saying that when I interpreted, I was "cruel" to her. During the therapy, Lecter disappeared, but later appeared again. This happened when the patient began to feel the lack of sufficient care on my part and to have doubts whether the relationship with me could become a substitute for the relationship with her father.[4]

The hallucinated figure does not have to be an image of a deceased or fictitious person. A young patient with hysterical personality disorder hallucinated her living grandmother, who appeared to her in difficult moments. This patient also received the most care in her childhood from her grandmother. During the many months of this girl's stay in the hospital, her grandmother turned into a doctor, to whom the girl was strongly attached. The doctor appeared to her in a white dress and with a halo around her head. Both figures appeared to—as the patient herself called it—dissuade her from hurting herself. And they were often successful. The girl was not psychotic, she had no disturbed contact with reality, she knew that the figure she "saw" did not really exist, that she was neither a physical person nor a "soul" (the person she represented was alive after all). However, she spoke to this figure and was answered. This is an example of the fact that human behavior is more strongly determined by the emotional level than by the rational one. The mind of this girl tested reality to a sufficient degree, but the need for contact was so great that its judgments were irrelevant. After some time, the patient realized that the living doctor was not as devoted to her as she had initially thought. And yet the figure did not cease to exist for her, she continued to fulfill her supporting function. It was only with time that she changed her dress to black and disappeared more often. The patient began to feel her loneliness more and more.

## Memory—Hallucination—the Figure

We can assume—as Jung did—that hallucinated "spirits" are essentially projections of the unconscious and autonomic complexes of our psyche (Jung 1990, 167). With the death of a loved one, the whole of affective investment loses its object, and thus partially goes to the unconscious system. At the same time, psychic contents and affections, which until now could take place within the relationship, and thus be kept as if away from the subject, begin to demand direct acceptance. When this is not possible, when the *ego* defends itself, repressing painful and difficult content, it returns in the projection form of hallucination. The hallucination becomes a substitute for the relationship and allows to exteriorize the conflicting aspects of personality. At the core of psychological problems that arise after the death of a loved one lies the fact that the cohesion of the psyche is relative. The sense of the coherent *ego* is sustained by the network of references to the outside world and people, and the system of ideas ("of oneself"). To keep a part of the psyche *coiled up*, the other one remains in *participation.*[5] This relation is clearly visible in the case of obsessive-compulsive disorder, anorexia, or symbiotic personalities (the phenomena discussed here most often concern the latter, i.e., the people who are mentally dependent on parents). The *coiling up* mechanism also takes part in the production of hallucinations—it produces compact and personified entities ("spirits," "specters"), because dialogue with these parts of the psyche is only possible in this form.

The author of the so-called psychophysics, Gustav Theodor Fechner, is also the author of an extremely interesting concept that goes further than Jung's theory of complexes. This is what Fechner wrote about ghosts of the dead:

> You have hitherto believed that the light form in which a dead person appears to you in remembrance is merely your own interior illusion. You are mistaken; it is itself a reality, which, with conscious step, not only comes to you but enters into you. (Fechner 1904, 97–98)

> Doctors call them phantasms, hallucinations. So they are for the living, yet, at the same time, they are actual apparitions of the dead, as we call them. For though they be the weaker forms of memory in us, how should they not also be the more pronounced corresponding apparitions. Therefore, why still dispute whether they are the one or the other when they are at once both. And why be afraid of ghosts, when you do not fear the remembered forms within you which they already are? (Fechner 1904, 98–99)

Fechner believed that spirits are the "third stage" of existence, and that people's thoughts and mental achievements exist after their physical death in this form (it resembles the notion of morphic field or the concept of Akashic records). So if everyone agreed that Plato's figuratively understood "spirit" lives in contemporary Europeans, because Plato provided foundations for the later development of culture, Fechner would say that this is not only a metaphorical existence, but a real one. The "remnants" of Plato's thoughts and achievements merge with other remnants of corresponding significance and contents, forming conscious and autonomous entities while fighting for influence on the human mind.[6] The author wrote:

> Man does not often know from whence his thoughts come to him: he is seized with a longing, a foreboding, or a joy, which he is quite unable to account for; he is urged to a force of activity, or a voice warns him away from it, without his being conscious of any special cause. These are the visitations of spirits, which think and act in him from another center than his own. Their influence is even more manifest in us, when, in abnormal conditions (clairvoyance or mental disorder) the really mutual relation of dependence between them and us is determined in their favor, so that we only passively receive what flows into us from them, without return on our part. (Fechner 1904, 25–26)

Spirits maintain their existence through ideas, effects of actions, and human memory. The spirit is a part of the psyche of the living and an autonomous figure at the same time. This is the area in which the psyche participates. The existence of the spirit depends on our memory, but at the same time it goes beyond it. The spirit ultimately turns out to be stronger than the psyche of the living. Fechner's concept indicates the transitional status of the psyche, i.e., it is not possible to unambiguously distinguish between the subjective and the objective, between the "product of the mind" and the "independent being." Does this concept have any clinical application? It seems that it very well explains the phenomenon of the influence of spirits, which seems stronger than the influence of memory, but maybe it is not related to the souls of the deceased.

## Restitution of the Relationship with the Deceased

A common phenomenon in depression and some personality disorders is the "deceased" who "calls." It is usually a relative, friend, or acquaintance. The quality and intensity of this phenomenon is arranged along the continuum, which begins with suicidal thoughts in some way connected to the memory of the deceased, and ends with multi-sensory hallucinations, in which the figure of the dead appears and orders to "follow him." Most often it is a more or less distinct voice "in the head" saying the following sentences: "I am waiting for you," "Come to me" or an aggressive and direct one "Kill yourself!"

Such an imperative to leave this world may be the direct cause of self-destructive acts and suicide attempts. This phenomenon is associated with Freud's "deferred obedience" (Freud 1996c, 142–43),[7] which may occur after the death of a parent. Then the subject unconsciously submits to the earlier wishes of the deceased person. It looks as if the person after his death had more power over the child than during his lifetime. Generally speaking, this powerful mechanism occurs when the child is not able to become sufficiently autonomous. As long as the parent lived, his descendant dealt with excessive dependence in various ways. He could create aggressive fantasies, isolate himself, or rebel to some extent. He functioned fairly normally, as the problematic spheres of his psyche were placed within the relationship. However, the parent did not give the child the opportunity to interiorize psychic skills, kept them with him, being unable to pass them on to his child (a common example is a mother who constantly criticizes the child's activities, requires resourcefulness, shows she is a role model, but in fact, she makes sure that the child will not learn anything from her). The descendant in turn avoided the awareness that he was unable to live independently. Although everything he did resulted from symbiosis with his parent, he deluded himself that he was driven by his free *ego*. However, he was not prepared for independent living, and his parent, so to speak, took certain psychological skills necessary for normal functioning with him to the grave. It can be said that this person was deprived of a "part" of the psyche when the relationship with the parent ended. Although the repertoire of possible behaviors is enormous, there are at least two types of the parent's activities that lead to such a situation. These activities are, on the one hand, the explicit exploitation and oppressing of the child, and on the other hand—overprotection described above, which is by no means an excess of love, but its distortion.

After the death of such a parent, there is emotional chaos, filled with fears of the future and strong affects, which—although formed within the relationship with the parent—only now begin to manifest themselves. The sense of guilt is probably the most common among these experiences. The person reproaches himself for having had aggressive impulses toward the dead parent. He does not feel that he can live for himself, free himself from the parent's influence. Because the parent never gave himself to him in a healthy and sufficient way, he constantly needs him. The psyche, so far dependent on him, tries to maintain the relationship with it, which is why it reconstructs the parent in itself. The individual, unable to be mentally independent, unconsciously "calls the spirit of the parent." Of course, such a strong attachment to the image of the deceased person must have negative consequences.

We will take a closer look at this process based on the case of a woman who was sexually abused by her father when she was a child. From the beginning, physical closeness between her and her father exceeded the normal parent-child relationship. From an early age she slept with him in one bed and was touched by him, which she treated as signs of usual closeness. Living with her father, the girl always had everything she needed, and he never shouted at her, he taught her and raised her. When she grew up, she sensed that there was something wrong about this relationship. The woman remembered that she had often tried to make him lose his temper, wanted him to get angry with her, to shout at her. Perhaps she expected that their relationship would be more lucid—the father would turn out to be bad and she would be able to isolate herself from him. It did not happen, however. This situation became the cause of a bond that is impossible to disentangle, just like the Gordian knot.

The father's complex, his "spirit" in her, caused her to destroy everything that could be her individual life and happiness. In this way she could be back in the "relationship" with her father. During the psychotherapy, there was a situation where the patient experienced me as competing with her father. This evoked a sense of loyalty to the father, who in some ways "stopped" her from making progress in the therapy and from living a normal life. When the patient imagined that someone was sitting in the empty chair in front of her, she felt his sinister and fascinating presence.

Here is another example—a case of a young, intelligent, and psychologically perceptive woman whose life was a series of unpleasant events caused by her parents. When she was a child, the parents were constantly arguing and during the arguments they set each other against her. According to her, they also acted jointly when they beat or otherwise mistreated her. She remembered she had been put in an old washing machine filled with water or beaten with an iron. For many years, the mother wrote a note in her diary: "Love your mother while she's with you, because it'll be too late when she's in the grave." She kept talking about death ("even when she was making pasta"), about the end of the world. Over and over again, the girl had to look at the photo album with the pictures of her grandmother's funeral or go with her mother to the cemetery, where she showed her graves of children.

The mother's behavior indicates what I have said above—the fear of death, which is ceded to the child. The mother, burdening the child—the being driven towards life and not knowing the realness of death—with the issue of death, wants to reduce her own fear of it. Although this patient could not say why she loved her father or mother, her serious psychological problems—depression, suicidal thoughts and hallucinations—began just after her mother's death (her father had died earlier). When the mother was dying, lying unconscious on a respirator, the daughter felt as if the mother reproached her. After her mother's death, she began to have olfactory and auditory hallucinations and delusions of influence. She had an impression that she could smell gasoline and coffee, hear her mother's ventilator-supported breathing. She associated "gasoline" with holidays, during which she and her parents had an accident, and "coffee"—with the morning coffee she made as a child for her mother (the mother shouted "you whore, hurry up," and she—though she did not know what "whore" meant—wanted to throw the cup at the mother). All these hallucinations are connected with the wish for the death of the mother and the resulting feeling of guilt (gasoline—the accident in which her mother could die; coffee—aggressive impulses toward her; breathing—anticipation of her death). The sense of responsibility for the mother's life had its origins also in other events. The child intervened several times during her suicide attempts and vicious family quarrels.

The patient did not want to be like her mother, but she felt that she became similar to her (her husband told her that she sometimes screamed like her). After the mother's death, two moles appeared on her face, exactly where her mother had had them. She did not go to her grave, and explained: "She is not there; what is there is bones and worms." Soon, she began to have delusions of influence and feel that she had an "open head," as if her mother had "wanted to get" to her head. During the therapy she said, "Why can't I break away from my mother? Now I know that my mother and I are in me and that we fight with each other." Through identification (reconstruction of the mother's personality aspects in her own *self*), the patient "raised her mother from the dead." In this way, she defended herself against the feeling of abandonment and guilt. It weakened when the mother remained "alive." It is a syndrome that occurs in many cases—a child wants to be completely different from a hurting parent but, because of such an attitude, feels even more abandoned by the parent and thus identifies with and becomes similar to him or her. In this way, the child in some way reconstructs the parent in him- or herself, making the child feel less lonely.

The phenomena of such restitution of the loved object take place in many ways. Someone may become like the parent, and someone else may be in a phantasmatic relationship with him. Some woman constantly made bad choices, from buying curtains to marriage—in this way she remained in an intimate relationship with her mother, who even after her death criticized the daughter's helplessness and the disastrous results of her teenage rebellion. It can also take the form of more massive transference, whose screen is society, institutions, and the whole environment as well as the person's lifestyle. A man organizes his life and perceives the world around him as if he were in relation to a loved one (a caretaker from childhood). To give an example, a patient with avoidant personality disorder who lived and perceived the world as if it had been about his mother. He was unable to undertake a job, or even look for it, because he perceived the existence of the labor market as lack of absolute maternal love. He constantly evaded the requirements of reality, because he could not agree to the fact that one must first try and show initiative, and only after that one can get acceptance and benefit. He felt aggrieved and misunderstood by the environment. He perceived all its demands and comments as a rejection and reason to withdraw from life even more. As a child, he felt his mother's lack of interest and understanding, she was also dissatis-fied with his attitude. She blamed the child for their bad relationship, not tak-ing into account that she had hurt him, giving him away to his grandmother for the first six years of his life.[8] The mother constantly expected something, not giving the boy absolute maternal acceptance. On this basis, an aversion to any requirements or even feedback developed in the child. Of course, the man's attitude should not be seen just as a passive remnant of his childhood. Deep in himself, this man wanted to function as he did. Through his attitude to the world, he reconstructed his relationship with his mother and, in this extraordinary way, defended himself against the fact that she was missing.

Another man's attitude towards life can be expressed by his childhood memory: he is lying in bed, looking fearfully into the dark room; his mother is lying behind him, giving him a sense of security. This man did not have suf-ficient maternal care in his childhood and strongly experienced the Oedipal conflict. His entire life—relationships, career—could be seen as an attempt to have the "mother behind his back" and keep her away from the "father." Although both his parents died long ago, during the psychotherapy he clearly felt that everything he did, he did in order "not to lose his mother." He felt that when he took a certain attitude, he "had a mother," and when he pre-sented another one—he "lost" her. His life was devoid of energy and mean-ing, it had the status of a dark childhood room, which he feared. It was only a shell, under which he hid the "mother." He could not take this life seriously, "enter the dark room and turn on the light," because then he would lose the feeling that his mother was close.

It is difficult for us to accept the fact that the deceased does not exist any longer, if he was a close person (had an influence on our mental life). Neu-rotic people very often internally refuse to accept the loss of relatives, which makes them experience their "existence" in various ways. Of course, they rationally and declaratively know perfectly well that the loved one has died, but some ways of their experiencing contradict this awareness. One woman, returning from her husband's funeral, caught herself thinking she could hardly wait to, finally . . . share the impressions of this ceremony with him. The next one, for a dozen or so years, left the light on at night, fearing that her late father would "come." Another patient could not empty the handbag of her late mother who in her childhood had tyrannized her, irrationally fear-ing her scream. Many years after her mother's death, when she experienced something that her mother would not have approved of, she spoke with a clear reproach: "Why is she silent now, why isn't she screaming?"—as if she had a grudge against her mother for tricking her, because she had implied that she had everything under control, and yet she succumbed to the power of death. Another woman reproached her husband for dying, although she had tried so hard to be a good wife. To a certain degree she still believed he lived somewhere in the world and finally would come to apologize to her, and then they would start living harmoniously together. The confidence that a newborn child is the reincarnation of the one who died is similar. The guilt for the death of the child may play a role here. If a newborn is the "same" child as the lost one, the guilt will obviously diminish. However, a child raised in such an atmosphere will be hurt. If, in addition, the child's gender is different from the sex of the child that died and the parents want to see the lost one in their new son or daughter, the child may develop gender identity issues. These states of pathological grief, experienced as various forms of denial of the loss of the loved one, without a doubt can be defined as a hidden cult of the dead.

## SELF-DESTRUCTION. THE
## PHANTASMS OF POWER, IMMORTALITY AND CARE

### Suicide Attempts

Individual immortality is a leitmotiv of many religions. Perhaps a few dozen thousand years ago the Neanderthals did not accept the prospect of the end of their individual existence. Their structured burials could attest to it (Szyjewski 2001, 201–5). It is possible that a burial is a manifestation of confidence or premonition that the existence of the deceased man has not come to a complete end. Otherwise, there would be no special need to handle his body in a special way. The idea, or perhaps a kind of feeling, of immortality seems to be deeply rooted in the psyche. In mental disorders, we often encounter both the increased fear of death and the belief in immortality or a kind of desire to die.

We will now deal with self-destructive behavior in the form of so-called "suicide attempts" to show that this behavior concerns unusual and specific phantasms (hidden attitudes and perceptions) related to death and life after death. Suicide attempts need to be distinguished from suicides—in the case of attempts we have the opportunity to analyze the motives and feelings of the person based on his own account. Often, these attempts are repeated, and the person is rescued not only by chance, but also owing to the circumstances of the suicide attempt (presence of relatives, physician, etc.). However, this type of act should not be underestimated, and calling it "manipulation of the environment" is not justified. Although it is not usually undertaken as an expression of the final decision to cease existence, it should not be understood as simple manipulation, because it is not subject to fully conscious control. We must understand that there is no contradiction in the fact that, notwithstanding the evident self-destructive impulses, a person to some extent protects himself, arranging the whole situation in a certain way (sometimes, in spite of this, another "attempt" becomes the last). It may happen that a psychiatrist, who is irritated by the repeated intoxication of his patient, says: "If you really wanted to kill yourself, you would have done it long ago" (I would not call it a form of psychotherapeutic paradoxical intervention, rather a manifestation of helplessness and aggression). In such a situation the patient feels completely rejected—he is, after all, scolded for still having a bit of faith in life, and no man should be faulted for it. These people have neither irrevocably decided to die, nor do they just deliberately manipulate the others. It is difficult to even say that their motive is somewhere in the middle, because it seems to be a superposition of both these possibilities. The classic, bivalent logic ceases to be enough when we want to penetrate into the more fundamental structures of the patient's motivation.

## Self-Destruction and the *Core Ego*

The suicidal patient had certain experiences that caused him to commit this self-destructive act.[9] As a result of frustration, pain, lack of understanding, and inner weakness, he withdrew and isolated his own *ego* from the world. He rejected everything that made him suffer. However, it still pressed on him—in the form of requirements of the world, emotions, memory, sense of guilt, or frustration. That is why, the external events along with his emotions, feelings, memories or plans had to join the rejected sphere. He therefore rejected everything that was outside the *ego*, and his *ego* became a *core ego*, more and more engulfed only in itself. However, that was not enough. The *non-ego* was still pushing, so the *core ego*, to protect its cohesion, had to counteract it. To remain locked in the *core ego*, the man raised his hand to everything that surrounded it. Including his biological existence.

The *ego*, withdrawing from life it cannot stand anymore, closes in itself. However, in the cases we address here, this process cannot reach a permanent end. The individual falls into a narrowing spiral, feeling that he can save himself only if he destroys everything that is beyond his *ego*. Therefore, it is not entirely correct to say that someone wants to "kill themselves"—perhaps man is not able to do this and "never kills himself," he never negates himself at his core. Rather, it is the *ego*, isolated in its last bastion, that passes judgment on the rest of the personality.

In cases of self-destruction, the *ego* does not accept self-limitedness and weakness. A self-destructive person establishes a power zone in himself, which is the *core ego*. This *ego* transcends everything that is weak in the individual. Because this "condensed" *ego* becomes the carrier of the entire identity of the individual, it can take the liberty of attacking the rest of the personality, without the paralyzing fear flowing from the self-preservation drive. This fear does not appear, because the self-destructive action aims at strengthening the *ego*, and therefore the self-preservation drive does not intervene. In self-destructive behavior, the person wants to reject from himself the sphere of life, which cannot be closed within the *ego* anymore. Adopting such an attitude is a way to gain a sense of power—only in the case of self-destruction can I create an area that I perceive as indestructible. When I sustain my life, I take care of myself and protect myself, soon I will see how weak I am in the face of fate. When I resist it, I cannot lose.

The *ego* of a healthy person contacts and controls the territories beyond it, constantly goes into the regions it cannot fully control. These regions are the body, parts of personality that participate in interpersonal relations and the requirements of the physical and social world. However, when problems arise, the *ego* can withdraw so much that it even diminishes its own limits. Anyone who has lived through an illness and physical suffering knows what this withdrawal of the *ego* is. In illness, the *ego* escapes from the body, perceives it as alien. It evades thinking, planning, lust. The area, which the subject recognizes as himself, shrinks. Freud, analyzing the life of a newborn, or the period of the *ego* formation, says:

> The tendency arises to dissociate from the ego everything which can give rise to pain, to cast it out and create a pure pleasure-ego, in contrast to a threatening outside, not-self. (Freud 2016, 3)

The "shrinking" force would lie at the very foundation of the *ego*, it would even be its driving force, the creator. The *ego* shrinks to stay happy, to keep itself for itself, not to give up its rule.

The so-called rites of passage, *rite de passage*, practiced in primitive cultures, are said to have a function that restores life (Leeuw 1997, 177–78). Perhaps the basis for their formation are the same psychological mechanisms as those we find in self-destruction in the form of self-mutilation. Paradoxically, by weakening the body (cutting, amputation of fingers, flogging, etc.) these ritual acts are supposed to give man more power. The man seeks to increase his own potency—I know I will not avoid being wounded by fate, so I become a fate for myself and wound myself. By taking control over the situation, my sense of security increases. And by getting close to death, it becomes possible for me to look at a new life.

### The Phantasm of Immortality

Man is a very strange being; his thought does not recognize any limitations in time or space. It is not true that we cannot imagine infinity, for it is quite the contrary—we cannot accept finitude and limitedness. The vision of finitude, to stay in our mind, must be actively sustained, as it is constantly pushed away by the spontaneous feeling of infinity. A child told that something happened before his birth and before he was "in Mommy's belly" will not understand the idea of his non-existence and will ask where he was then.

Physicists—like Stephen Hawking—go further and construct the cosmology of a "boundless universe" that is neither eternal nor has a beginning, because normally understood time does not apply to it at all (Hawking 1995, 144–80). It seems, however, that the intuitive thought opposes the recognition of such patterns and constantly goes beyond the boundless universe. Perhaps physicists themselves think in a similar way, only that, overwhelmed by mathematics, they do not trouble themselves with it.

In my opinion, a suicide can act under the influence of this sense of infinity and the phantasm of immortality. He often does not intend to simply "cease to exist," because his plans are more developed, so to speak. When he thinks of the world after suicide, he usually is present in that world. For example, the reaction of the environment to his suicide may be so important to him, as if he could directly feel its effects. So in his thinking, he goes beyond his death and lives after it. The suicide may therefore not only think about the world after his act, but even *be* in it. Just like a person who sacrifices his life for some idea or "future generations"—he reaps the rewards of his actions now. He "extends" his existence beyond death, "pulling" the effects of his deed to the present moment. Fantasies of one's own funeral in people who do not intend to kill themselves have a similar function. They want to see—here we can refer to Lacan—the enigma of the Other's desire, which is expressed in seeking an answer to the question: "How will my loved ones react to my disappearance?" (see Žižek 1997, 42).

## The Phantasm of the Guardian and the Supports of Existence

A person who attempts suicides and acts of self-destruction constantly experiments with his mortality and existential freedom. He tries to find an Archimedean point of support for existence, which, to his mind, cannot be suspended in the vacuum of freedom. He senses that he walks on the edge, but tries to prove to himself that he does not. He cannot come to terms with the fact that, ultimately, whether he will continue to live depends on his gesture. He is terrified by the fact that such an important decision is left to him. He wishes depriving himself of life was not so easy. He wishes there was someone or something that could be a barrier to his actions.

There is also a continuum here. Initially, the individual can expect some kind of support, interest, and help from other people. Then he secures himself, organizes his act in such a way that he can be rescued. He wants to reject his problems, forget about difficulties, cut himself off from responsibility, and at the same time get under the care of other people. When the despair grows, he basically does not believe that human help is possible any longer. And yet the need for care remains. Except that the ordinary caretaker becomes a phantasmatic figure. The man rejects the life that he has to actively support himself, because he wants an existence protected from the outside. Suicidal actions are like attempts to extort interference from the "supernatural force" that will support existence. This is a call for a *guardian* who will take away the suicide's ability to make such a destructive decision about his fate.

Therefore, an attempt to kill oneself may be an expression of the desire to be cared for and to reject the life that requires one's own care. Thus, the attempt may be motivated by the desire to reject what is tiring, but also by the desire to obtain something—the satisfaction of the need for care and sense of security.[10] The fantasy of the person who takes this path consists in identifying the rejection of self-care with obtaining care from the outside. It is an insane state in which it seems that if one loses more and more, at some point he will gain everything. And in case no one is watching, if everyone is so far away, the act becomes more and more extreme to make someone look. Even if it was someone who does not exist.

## The Denial of Mortality

In many mutilating or attempting-suicide people, the full awareness of death seems to be limited.[11] The person reaches the stage where benefits can only be achieved on the threshold of death, or rather "right beyond it." Therefore, he does not accept the fact that there is nothing of his previous life beyond this threshold. People who repeatedly undertake very serious attempts at suicide may be very intelligent, but their sense of the realness of death is incomplete. They show a severe impairment that is common to all of us: they cannot realize the realness of death because they do not want to accept their mortality. Here is a fragment of a patient's account describing her suicidal fantasy: "Then I'll kill myself with a knife and cover myself in bed. In the morning someone will come in, will say 'wake up,' will shake me, will finally uncover the quilt and will see the terrifying view." The language error, involving the use of the impossible sequence of actions, was probably not a coincidence. I also observed similar errors in other patients. Of course, the aforementioned woman was aware of the fact that she was mortal, but a closer analysis of her behavior and statements indicated that her psyche negated this seemingly obvious fact.

People with self-destructive behaviors are afraid of death and at the same time approach it. The more apparent their mortality seems to be, the closer they get to it, as if the maximum closeness could—as it does in the case of visual perception—blur the clear contours. People thinking about suicide can say that they are afraid they will "fail," that instead of losing their lives they will become invalids. This kind of "problem" is a denial of death, an expression of disbelief in its realness. These people, in fact, delude themselves with the vision of the indestructibility of life (which at most can be damaged). It also happens that neurotics discourse on their fears of a possible "awakening" in a buried coffin. The function of these fears is identical. Ignorance or underestimation of the possibility of death is obviously typical of a child. At first, the child does not know death at all, but even when he or she knows it, it may seem to be something not entirely real, something that does not concern the child. Becoming more and more aware of one's mortality is a process that can take a very long time, and which may end only in the face of death.

## IS THERE A SOUL?

### The Pathological Spiritualization

A "soul" is a postulated entity that is supposed to be a carrier of identity and permanent existence independent of the existence of the body. It should be noted that such an idea is constructed based on many phenomena in the field of psychology, psychopathology, and parapsychology, which do not necessarily confirm the ontic existence of the "soul." These phenomena include dreams,[12] hallucinations of the deceased, and pathological grief described above (in the form of fear of an assumed influence of a dead person), dissociative states (possession that seems to confirm the possible existence of a "spiritual being"; mediumic phenomena). Also the sense of an irreparable loss, for example in a situation of losing a child, causes that only faith in immaterial personality continuance makes it possible to cope with the pain. The woman's desire that her next child be a kind of undoing her previous miscarriage supports the image of the soul and its transmigration from the body of one child to another.

In people who, during childhood, experienced severe traumas such as mistreatment or sexual abuse, there is often a disturbed attitude towards their own body. These people can experience various sensations related to the distinction between "soul" and "body." So they may "not feel" their body, feel that they "are in the head," find the body disgusting and want to escape from it, they can also experience the sensation of exteriorization (the feeling that their consciousness separates from the body). All these phenomena are forms of defense against confrontation with the sphere of the body, which is the way to deeply hidden, negative emotions. Such people live their "soul," which means that they identify themselves with their mind and thinking, denying and rejecting the body. The distinction between the soul and the body is particularly clear to them. We can say that in their case the soul must be something existing, so that they can deal with difficult emotions, reject unacceptable areas of their person, and at the same time keep their identity. We have a similar situation in the case of anorexia. There is also an escape from the body, even an attempt to "be a soul."

Schizophrenia reveals similar elements, which in psychiatry even obtained a separate name: spiritualization (however, all the phenomena mentioned above can be described with this name, as "pathological spiritualization"). The schizophrenic's *ego* is afraid of people and reality with which it has less and less contact. In place of the real world, which can be influenced only through a holistic involvement, the ill person builds a world of fantasy that can be created even by the weak, withdrawn from the world *ego*. The schizophrenic's isolated *ego* becomes so ethereal that it may seem to the patient that he is a soul, a spirit, or God. The world and the sense of oneself seem to be losing their realness. One patient constantly talked about his incorporeality, he wondered if his hand would penetrate through another person, he fantasized about the incorporeal existence of people. He stuck a knife in his chest to "check if there would be blood" or if he was "already a soul." At the same time, he was afraid of knives and the fact that he could hurt somebody. Because he felt self-destructive impulses, partly manifested by the voices telling him to kill himself, his fantasies of incorporeality played a defensive role. He was afraid of his own and others' aggression, and with his incorporeality he wanted to secure himself and others.

## OBE, NDE, and Self-Observation

Parapsychology recognizes a phenomenon called *Out-of-Body Experience* (OBE), i.e., the so-called exteriorization. It is described as a state in which one experiences the existence of his consciousness as independent of the body. It can observe the body from various perspectives, just like one observes objects and other people (Bugaj 1990, 22). There are at least two variants of this state. The first, when the consciousness connected with the body disappears, and there is the consciousness associated with some place in space (e.g., the person looks at his body lying on the bed from the opposite corner of the room), and the second variant, where the consciousness of the subject is *equally* connected with the body and another place (from which it can observe the body as in the first example). Another phenomenon in which similar sensations occur is the *Near-Death Experience* (NDE), scientifically described for the first time by Raymond Moody (Moody 2015). Such phenomena are a strong premise for recognizing the possibility of "out-of-body existence."

Without trying to reduce these phenomena to disorders, we need to point out the clear parallels we will find in the field of psychopathology. Among the people diagnosed with depersonalization/derealization disorder (from the category of dissociative disorders) there are those whose experiences occur in OBE and NDE, although they are not related to such specific factors as a threat to life or meditation. One of them describes her experiences:

> I'll be standing behind my counter and, all of a sudden, I'm also standing a couple of feet away. I seem to be looking over my own shoulder as I'm talking with my customer. And in my head I'm commenting to myself on my own actions, as if I were a different person I was watching. Stuff like "Now she'll have to call the assistant manager to get approval for this transfer of funds." (Morrison 2014, 238)

In this context, we must take into account the already described pathological intensification of self-observation in narcissism. The narcissistic person may have the impression that he is looking at himself from the outside, or that both perspectives—the normal and that "from the side"—overlap. So in narcissism, there are very similar phenomena to those that occur in exteriorization and near-death states. Is it, then, that exteriorization is nothing more than the impression in people with narcissistic personality disorder? Or is it—which seems to be a daring hypothesis—that the physical ("astral") factor that is the basis of the "external eye" is exteriorized in narcissism? I do not think that the answer is that simple, however, in my opinion, the phenomenological convergences mean something.

## The Soul as a Result of the Need to Meet

Reflecting on the question of the "soul," we can also raise the issue of a relationship and meeting. Everyone enters a direct relationship with the other in a "psychophysical" way, that is, not only with the mind but also with the body. Of course, this is particularly evident in a sexual relationship. In the case of a meeting between a man and a woman (in a heterosexual relationship), the body becomes the basic source of information about the other, we infer whether someone is attractive to us from his body appearance. Body shape, facial features become the basis for extensive (partially formed unconsciously) judgments, opinions, as well as hopes and expectations. Hands, mouth, and eyes, shoulders, or buttocks become the construction material of the vision of the "personality" and "nature" of the partner, which determines the assessment more than the internal factors that are difficult to capture. The other person usually sees themselves differently. They associate their masculinity or femininity, and certainly their personal identity, with some external feature of the body to a definitely lesser extent than the external observer.

We have now come to an important moment: there is a discrepancy, no correspondence between the perspectives of both partners in the relationship. The internal perspective is always more "spiritualistic" and the external "psychosomatic." It is natural because a person must remain themselves for themselves, even if they lose their beauty or hand, and will no longer be the embodiment of masculinity, femininity, or anything else for the partner. However, if there are these two perspectives, then each meeting is something dynamic, if not risky. Others read us differently than we do because they perceive us from another place. They also have different expectations from us than we have from ourselves.

Let us analyze the example of a sexual meeting a bit more. A girl that someone compliments, saying that she has an amazing back and waist, can feel happy because of the affirmation of her femininity. Soon, the admirer can discover and underline the beauty of her mouth and hair, and all this—thanks to her feeling that she is noticed and appreciated—becomes a step towards a sexual relationship. However, this girl might as well be terrified of such a course of events. From this perspective, her body becomes a veil, a barrier that does not let the other look inside (his eye may not want to reach deeper anyway). She could feel that the partner's perception tells her to play a role that is not her role at all. She could see that their meeting, so intimate, it would seem, is in fact shallow, full of pretense, illusions, and superficiality. Everything will depend on whether she identifies with the external "psychosomatic" perspective or adopts an extremely "spiritualistic" attitude.

Most young people take an attitude close to the "psychosomatic" pole— they do not feel the stratification of perspectives yet, because their inner identity needs a strong external foundation. They want to be what others see in them, and it still seems to them that it is possible. It is not a fully mature attitude, but it is perfectly normal. On the other hand, there are people who are terrified, in a pathological way, of such an attitude. If our hypothetical girl belonged to their category, then every compliment and every affirmation of her corporeality or exterior would be stopped by her, she would have one counter-argument against everything: "This is not about me." She would be afraid that the meeting with the other takes place in the "psychosomatic" sphere, and not in the "spiritualistic" one—that it is not a meeting of souls, but more a meeting of bodies. It would be the fear of falsehood and the superficiality of the relationship. The elements of this dynamics often occur in anorexia. They are also characteristic of a personality with hysterical features.

The mentioned conflict in the situation of a meeting, which always takes place on two different levels, is unavoidable. In a meeting, both perspectives interact with each other, which implies constant tension. This, in turn, may involve attempts to relieve it by choosing one of the poles. One can identify with the "psychosomatic" perspective, although it would mean a kind of immaturity ("I am the way I look"), or demand from others that they look at them from the fully "spiritualistic" position ("I am not what you see"), which would be unrealistic. Both solutions would be an attempt to control the relationship. From the psychopathological view, the "psychosomatic" perspective is used by well-functioning and compensated narcissistic persons, and the "spiritualistic" one by narcissistic persons who do not function well, anorexics and some persons who were abused or neglected.

## AGAINST LIFE-TOWARDS-DEATH

### The Life Game

Blaise Pascal showed his psychological perceptiveness when he stated that the human inclination for amusements, games, and bustle is to help us escape from thinking about ourselves and, above all, from the awareness of death (Pascal 2018, 39–40). What Pascal noticed only in relation to amusements can be transferred to a wider plane of life. To avoid the awareness of death we do not just use games and amusements, but we can also change our whole life into a game. The goal of the game is to construct an artificial reality, to separate ourselves from the realities of life.

A psychological game is a common phenomenon that underlies countless human behaviors. This was noted by Eric Berne, who described many universal game patterns that occur in our lives (Berne 2016). Although he claimed that a game isolates from closeness, in the book *Games People Play: The Psychology of Human Relationships*, he also described its positive aspects. Reportedly, however, he did it under the pressure of the publisher (Hay 2010, 193). It is now believed that any psychological game is a negative phenomenon that stands in the way of full interpersonal contact and the truth.

Games are present in psychopathological states as well as in "everyday life." A psychological game is both a game with oneself and an interpersonal game, and both these aspects are intertwined. There can be many types of games, and they are based not only on words, but also on behaviors. A frequent element of games is to evoke a sense of guilt. Someone who never complains, always looks as if he suffered. When asked what happened, he replies that he can handle it and that there is nothing to worry about. It is clear, however, that he blames everyone around him. He will never express emotions and reproach directly, because in an open discussion these could turn out to be inadequate, invented or provoked by his own attitude. And he has already organized the reality and divided it into "good suffering ones" and "evil oppressors," classifying himself among the first. He does not blame anyone directly; on the contrary, he demonstrates that he accepts fate and does not complain. He realizes, however, that in this way he will arouse a greater sense of guilt in the people around. Someone else says: "I can't understand you at all. I'm not saying I'm the only one who's right, but I just can't understand you." What can happen when someone says so? On the surface, he presents himself as a person ready for dialogue and learning about different views, but implicitly tries to make the interlocutor feel guilty and lower his self-esteem. He shows him that he is a person who cannot be understood, someone who thinks illogically, perhaps even someone strange. In this way, keeping the sense of "being fair," he also implicitly gives vent to his aggression.

One of the simplest patterns of the game is to stalemate. If "either way is bad," there is an illusion of unchanging existence, it protects against the awareness of the passage of time. The game makes the individual dissolve in the system of interpersonal connections and intrigues. The psychological game blears and obscures reality, introducing artificial problems and goals. It provides the opportunity to escape from oneself and the world, and reduces the unpleasant necessity to reflect on transience. Take an illustrative model: life without a game is like a straight line. When we walk along this line, our eyes see it in its entirety and we cannot have any doubts that somewhere in front of us it inevitably ends. This is a sad perspective. Life filled with the game is different. It resembles a line full of sharp turns and even loops, so sometimes we are turned sideways, and sometimes the end of our line is behind us. Of course, we constantly go in the same direction. However, our awareness of death is unclear, sometimes we behave as though death did not exist. Take, for example, a relationship between a woman and a man. Perhaps we see it too seldom, but many relationships are based more on a game than love. Love straightens the line of our lives—if we love, we know that we love a mortal being, which makes us feel our mortality as well. Loving people have only one way, it is the way that ends with death. They are immersed in their being-towards-death because they are together. One reminds the other of their mortality. The common attempt to escape this awareness is frequent changes of partners. By frequently changing partners, one can avoid contact with the existential sphere of the partner's life, and thus not contact his own existential problem. When people get to know each other, when they are in a casual relationship, they do not talk about death. And even if they do, it usually is *just* a conversation, without deep contact with their own mortality in the face of the partner's mortality. Therefore, they can keep these aspects of the human condition away from the consciousness, focusing on pleasure, consumption, fun, or cooperation. If they decided to live together, they would need to directly face the issue of death. However, thanks to the game, they can have an apparent intimacy, which on the one hand allows them to meet various needs, and on the other—helps them escape from the overwhelming awareness of death.

## Mental Disorders as Games

We can take many mental disorders as games that create a false reality and allow to adopt a phantasmatic attitude towards the world. Of course, they are not conscious games, they are often dramatic and destructive, and always, to a large extent, uncontrolled by the individual. What is characteristic of any mental pathology is that it isolates from reality, from here and now, from responsibility, ability to love and be understanding (leaving aside partial sensitivity and perceptiveness). Separating from the manifestations of the real process of life, it also isolates from death. The only question is whether it is a specific by-product of isolation or a pathogenic factor, the main motive of isolation.

If we assume that something that is a reference point of the whole life must influence its manifestations, we get the answer to this question: fear of death must be one of the basic causes of mental disorders. We can consider disorders as forms of isolation from the real flow of life, as attempts to create one's own universe. Its basic feature will be no death in it. In the case of many psychopathological phenomena, there is a clear mechanism to escape from the awareness of death. It can even be said that they are ways to encapsulate this awareness and the resulting fear. A disorder is a kind of intrapsychic game whose aim is to remove this existential fact from the consciousness.

Hypochondria is the most evident example. The hypochondriac is constantly worried about his health and fantasizes that his organism malfunctions, that he suffers from some hidden, underdiagnosed disease. For these reasons, he constantly visits doctors, undertakes examinations and treatment. In fact, he separates himself from the awareness of death. His doctor has only one answer to these complaints and fears: "You are healthy, your fears are unfounded, nothing bad is going to happen to you." And this is the hypochondriac's point. Of course, he does not need to hear these words, but he constantly provokes such a response. In this way, he protects his consciousness from the real answer: "Yes, you will die one day."

The creation of artificial reality probably occurs in every mental disorder. I described it based on the example of depression, where the ideal *ego* protects itself in the shell of self-accusations, rejecting any real judgment, and thus any possible change. It is similar with obsessive-compulsive disorder, in which the *ego* seeks isolation in its own world, away from the changing, unpredictable world. In the acts of self-destruction, the *ego* creates a world where it rules over death. In the course of anorexia nervosa, the world of biological dependence is rejected by the *ego* seeking freedom. In schizophrenia, man hallucinates entire worlds. A person with conversion disorder, manifesting itself for example in a difficulty in speaking or walking, will "fight" his illness as if it was a real problem, although he unconsciously created it himself. He will produce a virtual reality, splitting himself into the "fighting" part and the one that is "being fought." Subconsciously, however, he probably expects to gain full control over his problem, potentially being able to miraculously heal himself at any moment. In this way, from a "part of himself," he creates an "environment," his own world, enabling him to leave the unsatisfying real world.

We can see a similar aspect in drug addiction and alcoholism. These addictions create a "single problem"—an addict does not experience any other distractions or frustrations except for the problem of having or not having the active substance. In particular, narcotics bind all spheres of the individual's functioning, all his needs, feelings and emotions. When physical pain appears in a drug addict (e.g., tired muscle soreness), physiological hunger, or some unpleasant emotional state (sense of loneliness, interpersonal problems), it is immediately associated with drug craving. All problems, from bad mood to the need for belongingness, are solved by taking drugs, and getting them becomes the only real problem. Therefore, drug addiction (as well as alcoholism) is not just a "source of problems"—thanks to it, one can also gain something, namely, freedom from existential problems.

Another case of negation of the basic aspects of life is perversions. In perversion there is a tendency to perceive a sexual object as immortal. Perverse sexual behaviors always consist in a kind of fetishism and a relationship with the "partial object." The pervert admires a foot, age, specific body structure, or specific behavior of the object of his desire, but never the whole person. This happens, among other things, because he wants to avoid contact with mortality. In contrast to a specific person who can irretrievably die, the object of his desire is constantly reborn in thousands of copies. Perhaps because of this "eternity" of the fetish, perverts take an almost religious attitude towards these objects (see Chasseguet-Smirgel 1974, 351).

## The Blockade of Vitality—Fantasy of the Unchangeable Being

Death is a problem for every human being, but perhaps it is a special one for neurotics. Jung said that just as the young neurotic fears life, so the old one fears death. Indeed, "old" neurotics show a surprising increase in fear, even of a thought of death, which in their life naturally gets closer and closer. However, it is not that the "young neurotic" is simply afraid of life, not death. The "young one" is afraid of life-that-ends-with-death. He differs from the "old" only in that he potentially has more life ahead of him, and that is why his defenses may be different.

Neurotic people often cannot even listen about death, they begin to feel weak and fearful. As we have already said, they do not accept the clear awareness of the passing of life, and sometimes they do not accept the fact of death of their relatives and maintain the illusion that the husband, wife or one of the parents is still alive.[13] One woman once said, referring to a conversation with her friend who spoke about buying a tomb for five coffins: "Five times eighty centimeters, that's four meters down. . . . One, even if they wanted, wouldn't get out." This woman, after the death of her brother, experienced a huge fear of death, she went to regular treatments and medical examinations to almost ten physicians. Her way to deal with life-that-ends-with-death was typical of many neurotics: she killed her vitality, spontaneity, and pleasure, not to realize the process of changeability of life. This is the source of the, characteristic of neurasthenia (chronic fatigue, irritability, and inability to experience joy and pleasure) and neurotic depression, sensitivity to sounds (e.g., birds singing, children's laughter), aversion to sunny days and avoiding any changes. For these negated elements are manifestations of life. And since they prove its variability, they also testify to its transitoriness.

Patients sometimes ask: "Why cannot I be happy?," "Why do I get scared, when I am happy or have some pleasure?," "When I feel good, why do I automatically imagine that something bad will happen?" There is one answer: states of pleasure, joy, happiness confront us with life itself, and therefore also with its transitoriness. There is a specific kind of defense here: stifled vitality gives the illusion that it will never end. In accordance with the principle that "all good things must come to an end" a fantasy is constructed that "what is unpleasant lasts enormously long." A person starts to live as a "living dead," which causes a specific mixing (at the level of fantasy) of the state of life and death, which now seem to overlap, as if they penetrated each other and were not absolutely disconnected. This is where the neurotic fear of waking up in the coffin begins—since I am not alive now, perhaps I will not be dead after my death.

So whereas healthy functioning, facing people and the requirements of reality, encounters the fundamental truth that says that life ends with death, pathology gives the possibility to avoid this awareness. By making one distance from people, close themselves in their own world, it makes it possible to avoid the fear of one's own death and that of the loved ones. Looping life, making it impossible to choose, taking life energy away, it causes that the person does not see the passage of time.

It seems, however, that one cannot escape from the awareness of death. It returns in a camouflaged form of fear. Perhaps this symptom can be understood as a signal that says: "Though you isolate yourself, you will die anyway; in addition, you will not achieve anything or give anything to anyone; come to your senses!" One often has the impression that if fear did not exist, many people would resemble robots. They would love no one, they would not be creative, they would not think about themselves and others, and their lives would be good. It is different, however. When someone lives like that for a while, he falls into fear. It is the voice of the human spirit that calls for transgression.

## STRONGER THAN GOD—CLINICAL CASE STUDY

Agatha, as I will call her, was diagnosed with schizophrenia, but when I spoke to her—although she did not function well, and her way of being evoked the impression of an intellectual deficit—did not show evident schizophrenic symptoms. One could sense her distance, lack of creativity, emotional shallowness. The patient was as if constantly in herself, did not relate to the interlocutor. The problem she wanted to deal with was obsessive blasphemous thoughts. Agatha blasphemed against the Holy Spirit. She said she could not resist it since she had read in a catechism that blasphemy against the Third Person of God is a mortal sin.[14] She clearly indicated that she blasphemed in her mind "deliberately." However, she said she did not want to do it any longer.

Agatha lived with her aunt until she was six, her parents only visited her, which is why she never felt enough care from them. She remembered that, as a child, she had been left late in the after-school club. When she waited for her mother, a specific mechanism was activated: she was very afraid that the mother would not come, and at the same time she repeated in her mind that she wanted her not to come. She was afraid even more then. She twisted her teeth when she heard that they could fall out because of it, although of course she did not want to get rid of them. She also pressed her eye, and another time she looked directly at a light bulb, because she knew that it could cause trouble with eyesight. When she was in the after-school club, waiting for her father or mother, she was afraid that she would not notice them when they come. She said that their appearance at the door would be a moment, just a few seconds, so if she was turned back then, she could miss that moment. In the first class (the time when her parents took her back), she became very attached to her jump rope, which she used for ritualized gestures. She currently has a collection of jump ropes that give her a sense of security. If she has one of them with her and can look at it, she is not bored and feels that she does not need anybody.

It seems that Agatha lacked a sense of the existence of a good object, a caring person, but she probably did not have a sufficiently developed object permanence in general either.[15] Objects and persons did not have a stable existence, in a sense they existed only when looking at them. Hence the need for the entire supply of jump ropes, because the existence of one was not certain. The lack of a stable object resulted in the lack of sense of security. Agatha's self-destructive behaviors (pressing the eye, twisting her teeth, looking at the light bulb, repeating that the mother would not come) were meant to provide her with this feeling. In what way? Agatha, not believing in anyone's protection, tried to prove to herself that she did not need it, that she could survive even if she acted to the detriment of herself.

In Agatha's statements one could notice grandiosity and fantasies about omnipotence. She claimed that grass grew in her aunt's yard only when she thought about it; that when something interested her, it immediately became public. She said she often guessed which date would be mentioned by the radio announcer, that she guessed that some man was the son of her neighbor. We find this feature also in other statements, which seemingly were not grandiose. Agatha said that "as the only one" (she said it in a specific way) in physical education classes, she had "reduced physical fitness," and that she was affected by "very rare side effects" of her medications. Moreover, in her childhood, when she heard a prophecy from a strange woman, she herself gave the "dates of death" of several relatives, including her mother. When the year of her mother's supposed death came, she feared that her prophecy would come true (but in fact she was excited about the chance that her alleged skills could prove to be real).

Agatha confided that she thought she would never die, that her life would end only with the end of the entire cosmos. We should not interpret this feeling using a non-explanatory statement that it is a psychotic symptom.[16] This feeling is probably a consequence of non-relationality (emotional inability to enter into relationships), so Agatha's narcissism/autism. Man learns who he is only through contacts and relationships with others. The deeper his relations, the more he can learn about himself. If other people play a smaller and smaller role in our lives, the image of oneself begins to play a more and more important one. The realness of this image, in terms of its correspondence with reality, is inversely proportional to the degree of concentration on oneself. When others disappear from the area of our experience, experiencing oneself can become extremely untrue. One can even feel immortal. This mechanism probably underlay the fantasy of immortality, which afflicted some of the emperors and dictators. Ruling the lives of others, they did not stand on one plane with anyone. Nobody around was equal, so they could not learn any-thing from them, gain anything. They were so great and so lonely that they ceased to be able to imagine that they would face the same fate as all of their subjects.

It is characteristic that every thought of potential care became threatening to her. Why? Because if there is a guardian and a need for care, there is also a chance to be failed. That is why she tried to prove that such a need did not exist. It would be best to believe that there is no guardian. This mechanism was fully expressed in "blasphemy" against the Holy Spirit. Agatha tried to prove to herself that she would manage even if she committed a mortal sin, even if she cut herself off from God. Whereas most people would like God to exist, counting on his protection and consolation, she wished He had not existed. She was afraid that if God exists, He is severe and never forgives, giving only a guarantee of a painful punishment and confirming the exis-tence of hell. So in fact, through self-destructive behaviors and isolation, she wanted to negate the existence of God and almost become similar to Him. In order not to be at the mercy of God. She probably experienced her parents in a similar way—she wished they had not existed. Because at the time when she believed in them and counted on them, they let her down. On the other hand, Agatha "blasphemed" against God, she did not simply forget about Him. So she was in a relationship with Him. Apparently, she still needed relationships, also with her parents.

## NOTES

1. Quotation translated from Polish by Barbara Gąstoł.

2. In order to clarify this issue, I will refer to an analogy in the field of physiol-ogy—the biological stress concept developed by Hans Selye. Selye wondered why the majority of physical illnesses, regardless of the specificity of their image, manifest a certain group of non-specific, always occurring symptoms, which he called the Gen-eral Adaptation Syndrome (GAS). In addition, the Local Adaptation Syndrome oc-curs in the area directly affected by the injury, for example inflammation (the whole stress reaction consists of three factors: local effects of the stressor, the body's defen-sive response and factors inhibiting this response). The general adaptation syndrome, although it plays an important role in defending an organism that fights a pathogen, can become a "disease of adaptation" (see Selye 1960, 59–60). Similarly, in the case of mental disorders: there is a traumatic factor and a psychological response in the form of adaptation, which in general creates a psychopathological symptom, exter-nally perceived as bizarre and unnecessary. In some cases, this adaptation becomes a chronic condition, in which it is difficult to see the aspect of adaptation.

3. Imperative voices are a psychotic symptom; they mean that the patient "hears" commands addressed to him.

4. The hallucinations of strange faces were probably conditioned by a mechanism similar to the one that created Lecter—the "faces," except for the protective aspect, also had an aggressive side, manifesting it for instance in their demonic appearance. The creation of the "guardian-persecutor" was certainly not the only mechanism that produced these hallucinations. The projection of self-aggression could have been accompanied by the phenomenon of condensation, causing the image to include, for example, the figure of the patient herself (she was premature, she regressed to early childhood in some aspects, and the "face" looked just as the face of a newborn). This shows how complicated and ambiguous a hallucination can be.

5. *Participation* is not noticed, because looking at the psyche, we use cognitive categories arising in contact with the body and things, that is the objects with clearly defined spatial boundaries. This is responsible for sustaining the vision of the *ego* as having clear boundaries. However, such a picture turns out to be wrong as soon as we look closely at the functioning of neurotics, people with personality disorders or schizophrenia. My view on this matter corresponds with, for example, the remarks of Nietzsche, who contradicted the idea of the monadic subject (Nietzsche 2004a, 21, 35, 70), and with the assertions of Lacan considering the sense of the *ego* as an essentially phantasmatic product of the observation process of the body (Lacan 1987, 5-9).

6. At this point, Fechner's concept resembles the modern idea of memes ("units of cultural inheritance" which, like genes, are to fight for survival and reproduction).

7. Freud considers the phenomenon of deferred obedience also in relation to the origins of totemism: the murdered forefather gains the strength he did not have in his lifetime, his sons by exalting the totem animal, that is, his symbol and substitute, obey him. However, this situation may happen without the "historical" death of the father, and only as a result of the reaction to aggressive impulses towards him (Freud 2004).

8. From my observations, I conclude that one can speak of the "grandmother's child" syndrome. I often encounter people who—usually until the age of 6 or 7, that is, before going to school—lived and were brought up mainly by their grandmother (and the grandfather, although he, if he was present, usually played a supporting role). Sometimes they do not know why their parents were not with them, as the family did not talk about it. However, this biographical fact never goes unnoticed, no matter how caring and understanding the grandmother was. It is always encoded as rejection on the part of the parents, even if these emotions were hidden very deeply and clearly unconscious. If the child is raised by the grandmother he or she is often isolated from activity and more emotional manifestations of life. As adults, people brought up in this way hold a grudge against their parents. They are often avoidant, withdrawn, or experience other types of problems resulting from early deficits in closeness of the parents.

9. The self-destructive mechanisms described here are not the only ones and do not apply to all possible cases to the same extent. Perhaps, however, they concern quite a large group of people, in particular those who recurrently attempt to commit suicide. Many of them are diagnosed with emotionally unstable (*borderline*) personality disorder.

10. A suicidal act has an ambivalent meaning: although the person says he does not want any help, his behavior expresses helplessness and a cry for support and

relationship. However, he cannot admit even to himself that he needs others so badly. Although he says: "I do not care about my life," "I do not need any help," he involves the people around in his life through repeated suicide attempts. Each attempt brings him a strong "wave" of contact with other people (shock caused by finding the suicide, resuscitation or gastric lavage, and other procedures performed by teams of people), which he more or less consciously wants.

11. Self-mutilators (usually with *borderline* pathology) underestimate the likelihood of death more than those without a history of self-mutilation (Stanley, Gameroff, Michalsen, and Mann 2001, 427–32). In my opinion, the difference between the two groups may result from the fact that in the case of self-mutilators there is a phantasm of immortality, and "suicide," just as self-mutilation, serves as a game that isolates from the awareness of death.

12. The content of dreams, such as seeing the deceased or distant places, may suggest that a "soul" leaves the dreamer's body (the assumption of such reasoning in primitive peoples is the basis of Edward Burnett Tylor's animistic theory of religion).

13. According to Freud, the kind of thinking, which consists in tolerating two mutually exclusive contents (accepting that a given person has died, and at the same time hoping that he is still alive; accepting and not accepting at the same time) fully manifests itself in fetishism. The fetishist acknowledges, and at the same time denies the fact that the female has no penis. The fetish is just a substitute for this woman's (mother's) phallus. A little boy initially imagines that his mother has, like him, a penis. When he discovers that women do not have it, he experiences a strong fear (castration anxiety) that he too can lose his penis. Therefore, he must deny this fact and establish a representation of the "female penis" (hair, shoes, garments, etc.; Freud 2007, 303–9).

14. The so-called blasphemy against the Holy Spirit is regarded in the Church as the only sin that cannot be forgiven. This results from what Jesus said, "Therefore I say unto you, Every sin and blasphemy shall be forgiven unto men; but the blasphemy against the Spirit shall not be forgiven" (Mt 12:31). According to theology, this leads to a sin, in short, it is a fully conscious rejection of one's salvation or self-confidence that one will be saved despite all bad deeds.

15. The concept of object permanence is very important in Jean Piaget's theory of cognitive development of children. The physical object, as an invariant, is not an inborn idea, but is shaped in the process of a child's sensorimotor activity. Only the eight- to ten-month-old child starts searching for an object that is not within sight. Earlier, hidden objects ceased to exist for the infant (Wadsworth 1998, 58–59). The issue of permanence may be similar when it comes to a person, not an ordinary material object. One woman did a specific "experiment" in her childhood: when watching someone walking down the street, she stopped looking at them for a short moment then peeked to check if they were still moving at that time. She suspected that people may have stopped moving when she did not look at them. Also, she was afraid that her parents would not pick her up from kindergarten or that the mother would not find her if the girl left home.

16. One should also note that Agatha keeps her experiencing in some perspective. If she did not—as it can happen in psychosis—Agatha would not say that she "feels," that it "seems to her," etc., but that she simply "is" (immortal).

# Bibliography

Alanen, Yrjö O. 2000. *Schizofrenia. Jej przyczyny i leczenie dostosowane do potrzeb*, translated by Jacek Bomba. Warszawa: Instytut Psychiatrii i Neurologii.

Amorth, Gabriele. 1997. *Wyznania egzorcysty*, translated by Franciszek Gołębiowski. Częstochowa: Edycja Świętego Pawła.

———. 1999. *Egzorcyści i psychiatrzy*, translated by Witold Wiśniowski. Częstochowa: Edycja Świętego Pawła.

———. 2002. *Nowe wyznania egzorcysty*, translated by Władysława Zasiura. Częstochowa: Edycja Świętego Pawła.

Amorth, Gabriele, and Sławomir Sznurkowski. 2017. *Nie daj się zwyciężyć złu*. Częstochowa: Edycja Świętego Pawła.

Amyot, Fabienne. 2007. *Byłam opętana. Świadectwo uwolnienia przez egzorcyzm*, translated by Zofia Pająk. Kraków: Wydawnictwo eSPe.

Antonovsky, Aaron. 1995. *Rozwikłanie tajemnicy zdrowia. Jak radzić sobie ze stresem i pozostać zdrowym*, translated by Helena Grzegołowska–Klarkowska. Warszawa: Fundacja IPN.

Balthasar, Hans Urs von (ed.). 2001. *Origen, Spirit and Fire: A Thematic Anthology of His Writings*, translated by J. Daly. Washington: The Catholic University of America Press.

Barbaro, Bogdan de (ed.). 1999. *Schizofrenia w rodzinie*. Kraków: Wydawnictwo Uniwersytetu Jagiellońskiego.

Bateson, Gregory, Don D. Jackson, Jay Haley, and John Weakland. 1956. "Toward a Theory Of Schizophrenia." *Behavioral Science*. 1(4): 251–254.

Bednarczyk, Andrzej. 1999. *Medycyna i filozofia w starożytności*. Warszawa: Uniwersytet Warszawski, Wydział Filozofii i Socjologii.

Berne, Eric. 1973. *What Do You Say After You Say Hello?* New York: Bantam Books.

———. 2016. *Games People Play: The Psychology of Human Relationships*. London: Penguin.

Betts, Tim, and Sarah Boden. 1991. "Pseudoseizures (non-epileptic attack disorder)." In *Women and Epilepsy*, edited by M. Trimble, 243–58. New York: John Wiley and Sons.

Bloor, David. 1991. *Knowledge and Social Imagery*. Chicago and London: The University of Chicago Press.

Buck-Zerchin, Dorothea Sophie. 2000. "Medyczny model choroby w psychiatrii (środowiskowej) jako źródło cierpienia." *Dialog*, 9. Kraków—Münster.

Bugaj, Roman. 1990. *Eksterioryzacja—istnienie poza ciałem*. Warszawa: Wydawnictwo Czasopism i Książek Technicznych SIGMA NOT.

Bunyan, John. 1845. *The Life of John Bunyan*. London: Samuel Bagster and Sons.

Burchardt, Jerzy. 1979. *List Witelona do Ludwika we Lwówku Śląskim. Problematyka teoriopoznawcza, kosmologiczna i medyczna*. Wrocław: Zakład Narodowy im. Ossolińskich—Wydawnictwo Polskiej Akademii Nauk.

Buss, David M. 2016. *Evolutionary Psychology: The New Science of the Mind*. London, New York: Routledge.

Cardeña, Etzel. 2018. "The Experimental Evidence for Parapsychological Phenomena: A Review." *American Psychologist*, vol. 73 (5): 663–677.

Cavendish, Richard, and J. B. Rhine. 1992. *Świat tajemny. Leksykon magii, okultyzmu i parapsychologii*, translated by Stanisław Gogolewski, Barbara Lewandowska-Tomaszczyk, and Jerzy Tomaszczyk. Łódź: Wydawnictwo Łódzkie.

Chasseguet–Smirgel, Janine. 1974. "Perversion, Idealization and Sublimation." *International Journal of Psychoanalysis*, 55 (3): 349–357.

Chertok, Léon, and Ferdinand de Saussure. 1988. *Rewolucja psychoterapeutyczna. Od Mesmera do Freuda*, translated by Artur Kowaliszyn. Warszawa: Wydawnictwo Naukowe PWN.

Chiodo, Mariangela D'Onza. 2002. *Buddyzm*, translated by Krzysztof Stopa. Kraków: Wydawnictwo WAM.

Chudziński, Wojciech. 2013. *Channeling. Od chirurgów z zaświatów do "maszyn umysłu."* Bydgoszcz: Wydawnictwo "Arcanus."

Copernicus, Nicolaus. 1978. *On the Revolutions*, translated by Edward Rosen, edited by Jerzy Dobrzycki. Poland: Państwowe Wydawnictwo Naukowe, Great Britain: The Macmillian Press.

Dąbrowski, Kazimierz. 1979. *Dezintegracja pozytywna*. Warszawa: Państwowy Instytut Wydawniczy.

Dawkins, Richard. 2016a. *The Extended Phenotype: The Long Reach of the Gene*. Oxford: Oxford University Press.

———. 2016b. *The Selfish Gene*. Oxford: Oxford University Press.

Dianni, Jadwiga, and Adam Wachułka. 1963. *Tysiąc lat polskiej myśli matematycznej*. Warszawa: Państwowe Zakłady Wydawnictw Szkolnych.

Diogenes Laertius. 2018. *Lives of the Eminent Philosophers*, translated by Pamela Mensch, edited by James Miller. Oxford: Oxford University Press.

Dobroczyński, Bartłomiej. 2001. *Ciemna strona psychiki. Geneza i historia idei nieświadomości*. Kraków: Wydawnictwo Uniwersytetu Jagiellońskiego.

Drury, Nevill. 1995. *Psychologia transpersonalna. Ludzki potencjał*, translated by Henryk Smagacz. Poznań: Wydawnictwo Zysk i S-ka.

Dryjski, Albert. 1931. "Współczesne teorje podświadomości." *Kwartalnik Filozoficzny*, vol. 9. Kraków.

Dubrow, Aleksander, and Wieniamin Puszkin. 1989. *Parapsychologia a współczesne przyrodoznawstwo.* Warszawa: Krajowa Agencja Wydawnicza.

Dudek, Zenon Waldemar. 2002. *Podstawy psychologii Junga. Od psychologii głębi do psychologii integralnej.* Warszawa: ENETEIA.

Durkheim, Émile. 2008. *The Elementary Forms of the Religious Life*, translated by Joseph Ward Swain. Mineola, New York: Dover Publications.

Eisenbud, Jule. 1970. *PSI and Psychoanalysis: Studies in the Psychoanalysis of Psi-Conditioned Behavior.* New York: Grune & Stratton.

Eliade, Mircea. 1994a. *Historia wierzeń religijnych*, vol. 2, translated by Stanisław Tokarski. Warszawa: Instytut Wydawniczy PAX.

———. 1994b. *Szamanizm i archaiczne techniki ekstazy*, translated by Krzysztof Kocjan. Warszawa: Wydawnictwo Naukowe PWN.

Falala, Gerard, and Marie-Paule Florin. 1998. *Vademecum homeopatii*, translated by Anna Anczuków. Lublin: "Daimonion."

Fauman, Michael A. 1994. *Study Guide to DSM–IV.* Washington: American Psychiatric Press.

Fechner, Gustav Theodor. 1904. *The Little Book of Life After Death*, translated by Mary C. Wadsworth. Boston: Little, Brown, & Company.

Feuerbach, Ludwig. 1980. *Thoughts on Death and Immortality*, translated by James A. Massey. Berkeley, Los Angeles, London: University of California Press.

———. 2008. *The Essence of Christianity*, translated by George Eliot. Mineola, New York: Dover Publications.

———. 2017. *Lectures on the Essence of Religion*, translated by Ralph Manheim. Eugene: Wipf and Stock Publishers.

Fiore, Edith. 1995. *The Unquiet Dead: A Psychologist Treats Spirit Possession.* New York: Ballantine Books.

Fleck, Ludwik. 1979. *Genesis and Development of a Scientific Fact*, translated by Fred Bradley and Thaddeus J. Trenn, edited by Thaddeus J. Trenn and Robert K. Merton. Chicago, London: The University of Chicago.

Fontelle, Marc-Antoine. 2004. *Egzorcyzm w nauczaniu i posłudze Kościoła katolickiego*, translated by Jan Jędraszek. Ząbki: Apostolicum, Katowice: Księgarnia św. Jacka.

Frazer, George James. 1965. *Złota Gałąź*, translated by Henryk Krzeczkowski. Warszawa: Państwowy Instytut *Wydawniczy.*

Frenzel, Ivo. 1994. *Nietzsche*, translated by Jacek Dziubiński. Wrocław: Wydawnictwo Dolnośląskie.

Freud, Sigmund. 1933. *New Introductory Lectures on Psycho-Analysis.* New York: Carlton House.

———. 1938. "Three Contributions to the Theory of Sex." In *The Basic Writings of Sigmund Freud*, translated and edited by A. A. Brill, 553–629. New York: The Modern Library.

———. 1950. *Collected Papers*, vol. V, edited by James Strachey. London: The Hogarth Press.

————. 1957a. "Leonardo da Vinci and a memory of his Childhood." In *The Standard Edition of the Complete Psychological Works of Sigmund Freud*, translated and edited by James Strachey, vol. 11: 57–137. London: Hogarth Press.

————. 1957b. "On Narcissism: An Introduction." In *The Standard Edition of the Complete Psychological Works of Sigmund Freud*, translated and edited by James Strachey, vol. 14: 67–102. London: Hogarth Press.

————. 1961a. "A Seventeenth-Century Demonological Neurosis." In *The Standard Edition of the Complete Psychological Works of Sigmund Freud*, translated and edited by James Strachey, vol. 19: 67–106. London: Hogarth Press.

————. 1961b. "Future of an Illusion." In *The Standard Edition of the Complete Psychological Works of Sigmund Freud*, translated and edited by James Strachey, vol. 21: 1–56. London: Hogarth Press.

————. 1974. "Obsessive Actions and Religious Practices." In *The Standard Edition of the Complete Psychological Works of Sigmund Freud*, translated and edited by James Strachey, vol. 9: 117–27. London: Hogarth Press.

————. 1991. *Introductory Lectures on Psychoanalysis*, translated by James Strachey, edited by James Strachey and Angela Richards. London: Penguin Books.

————. 1996. "Uwagi na temat pewnego przypadku nerwicy natręctw," translated by Dariusz Rogalski. In *Charakter a erotyka*. Warszawa: Wydawnictwo KR.

————. 1997a. "Romans rodzinny neurotyków," translated by Robert Reszke. In *Pisma psychologiczne*. Warszawa: Wydawnictwo KR.

————. 1997b. "Przypadek wyleczenia hipnozą razem z uwagami o powstawaniu symptomów histerycznych przez 'opór'," In Ingrid Kästner, and Christina Schröder. *Zygmunt Freud (1856–1939). Badacz umysłu, neurolog, psychoterapeuta. Teksty wybrane*, translated by Bogumił Płonka, Bożena Płonka-Syroka, and Ryszard Ziobro. Wrocław: Wydawnictwo Arboretum.

————. 1997c. "Female Sexuality." In *Sexuality and The Psychology of Love*, edited by Philip Rieff, 184–201. New York: Touchstone.

————. 1997d. "Certain Neurotic Mechanisms in Jealousy, Paranoia, and Homosexuality." In *Sexuality and The Psychology of Love*, edited by Philip Rieff, 150–160. New York: Touchstone.

————. 2004. *Totem and Taboo. Some Points of Agreement between the Mental Lives of Savages and Neurotics*, translated by James Strachey. London, New York: Routledge.

————. 2007. "Fetyszyzm," translated by Robert Reszke. In *Psychologia nieświadomości*. Warszawa: Wydawnictwo KR.

————. 2016. *Civilization and Its Discontents*, translated by Joan Riviere, edited by Stanley Appelbaum (general editor), Thomas Crofts (editor of the volume). Mineola, New York: Dover Publications.

————. 2017. *Poza zasadą przyjemności*, translated by Jerzy Prokopiuk. Warszawa: Wydawnictwo Naukowe PWN.

Freud, Sigmund, and Josef Breuer. 2008. *Studia nad histerią*, translated by Robert Reszke, Warszawa: Wydawnictwo KR.

Frith, Chris, and Connie Cahill. 2001. "Zaburzenia psychotyczne: schizofrenia, psychozy afektywne i paranoja [Psychotic disturbances: schizophrenia, affective psychoses and paranoia]," translated by Jan Karłowski. In Arnold A. Lazarus, and Andrew M. Colman. *Psychopatologia.* Poznań: Wydawnictwo Zysk i S-ka.

Fromm, Erich. 1967. *Psychoanalysis and Religion.* New Haven, London: Yale University Press.

———. 1998. *Anatomia ludzkiej destrukcyjności,* translated by Jan Karłowski. Poznań: Rebis.

———. 1999. *Man for Himself: An Inquiry into the Psychology of Ethics.* Oxon: Routledge.

———. 2000a. *Psychoanaliza a religia,* translated by Jan Karłowski. Poznań: Rebis.

———. 2000b. *Zerwać okowy iluzji,* translated by Jan Karłowski. Poznań: Rebis.

———. 2000c. *Kryzys psychoanalizy,* translated by Wojsław Brydak. Poznań: Rebis.

Fromm, Erich, D. T Suzuki, and Richard De Martino. 2000. *Buddyzm zen i psychoanaliza,* translated by Marek Macko. Poznań: Rebis.

Furley, David. 1987. *The Greek Cosmologists: Volume 1, The Formation of the Atomic Theory and Its Earliest Critics.* Cambridge: Cambridge University Press.

Gabbard, Glen O. 2000. *Psychodynamic Psychiatry in Clinical Practice. The DSM – IV Edition.* Washington: American Psychiatric Press.

Goldstein, Eda G. 1990. *Borderline Disorders: Clinical Models and Techniques.* New York, London: The Guilford Press.

Graves, Robert. 2017. *The Greek Myths: The Complete and Definitive Edition.* London: Penguin Books.

Green, André, and Gregorio Kohon. 2005. *Love and Its Vicissitudes.* London, New York: Routledge.

Grof, Stanislav. 1985. *Beyond the Brain: Birth, Death, and Transcendence in Psychotherapy.* New York: State University of New York Press.

———. 1988. *The Adventure of Self-Discovery: Dimensions of Consciousness and New Perspectives in Psychotherapy and Inner Exploration.* New York: State University of New York Press.

———. 2010. *Kiedy niemożliwe staje się możliwe. Przygody z niezwykłymi stanami rzeczywistości,* translated by Maciej Lorenc, and Dariusz Misiuna. Warszawa: Okultura.

Grotstein, James S. 1999. "The alter ego i déjà vu phenomena." In *The Plural Self: Multiplicity in Everyday Life,* edited by John Rowan and Mick Cooper, 28-50. London, Thousand Oaks, New Delhi: Sage.

Grün, Anselm. 1998. *Post,* translated by The Benedictines of Tyniec. Kraków: Tyniec Wydawnictwo Benedyktynów.

Grzywa, Anna. 2000. *Omamy i urojenia.* Wrocław: Wydawnictwo Medyczne Urban & Partner.

Hart, Onno van der, and M. J. Dorahy. 2009. "History of the Concept of Dissociation." In *Dissociation and the Dissociative Disorders: DSM-V and Beyond,* edited by Paul F. Dell, and John A. O'Neil, 3-26. New York: Routledge.

Hawking, Stephen. 1995. *Ilustrowana krótka historia czasu,* translated by Piotr Amsterdamski. Poznań: Wydawnictwo Zysk i S-ka.

Hay, Julie. 2010. *Analiza transakcyjna dla trenerów,* translated by Ewelina Wójcik. Kraków: Grupa Doradczo-Szkoleniowa TRANSMISJA.

Heidel, Alexander. 1963. *The Babylonian Genesis: The Story of Creation.* Chicago, London: The University of Chicago Press.

Hellinger, Bert, Gunthard Weber, and Hunter Beaumont. 1998. *Love's Hidden Symmetry: What Makes Love Work in Relationships.* Phoenix: Zeig, Tucker & Co.

Hellinger, Bert, and Andrzej Nehrebecki. 2012. *Miłość zaklęta w chorobie.* Kraków: Wydawnictwo Pocieszka.

Hilgard, Ernest R. 1977. "The Problem of Divided Consciousness: A Neodissociation Interpretation." *Annals of The New York Academy of Sciences*, vol. 296: 48–59.

Hinshelwood, Robert Douglas. 1991. *A Dictionary of Kleinian Thought.* London: Free Association Books.

———. 1994. *Clinical Klein.* London: Free Association Books.

Hoevels, Fritz Erik. 1997. *Psychoanaliza i religia. Pisma zebrane*, translated by Wojciech Kunicki. Freiburg, Wrocław: Ahriman—International.

Höffe, Otfried. 1995. *Immanuel Kant*, translated by Andrzej Maciej Kaniowski. Warszawa: Wydawnictwo Naukowe PWN.

Hollingdale, R. J. 2001. *Nietzsche: The Man and His Philosophy.* Cambridge: Cambridge University Press.

Holy Bible: American Standard Version—New & Old Testament. 2018. Kindle.

Hoppál, Mihály. 2009. *Szamani eurazjatyccy*, translated by Agnieszka Barszczewska. Warszawa: Wydawnictwo Iskry.

Horney, Karen. 2000. *Wykłady ostatnie*, translated by Aleksander Gomola. Poznań: Dom Wydawniczy Rebis.

Hume, David. 2012. "An Enquiry Concerning Human Understanding." In *Classics of Western Philosophy*, edited by Steven M. Cahn, 834–899. Cambridge: Hackett Publishing Company.

Iwicka, Renata. 2017. *Źródła klasycznej demonologii japońskiej.* Kraków: Wydawnictwo Uniwersytetu Jagiellońskiego.

Jackowski, Krzysztof, and Krzysztof Janoszka. 2018. *Jasnowidz na policyjnym etacie.* Kraków: Wydawnictwo SQN.

Jacobi, Jolande. 1996. *Psychologia C. G. Junga*, translated by Stanisław Łypacewicz. Warszawa: Wydawnictwo Ewa Korczewska L.C.

Jaczynowska, Maria. 1987. *Religie świata rzymskiego.* Warszawa: Wydawnictwo Naukowe PWN.

Jakubik, Andrzej. 1979. *Histeria.* Warszawa: PZWL.

Jarosz, M. 2000. "Selektywność, biegunowość i cechy charakterystyczne schizofrenii autystycznej i syntonicznej." *Psychiatria Polska*, 34(5): 765–72.

Jonas, Hans. 1994. *Religia gnozy*, translated by Marek Klimowicz. Kraków: Platan.

Jung, Carl Gustav. 1964. *Man and His Symbols.* London: Aldus Books.

———. 1976. *The Collected Works of C. G. Jung, Volume 5: Symbols of Transformation: an Analysis of the Prelude to a Case of Schizophrenia*, translated by R. F. C. Hull, edited by William McGuire et al. Princeton: Princeton University Press.

———. 1980. *The Archetypes and the Collective Unconscious*, translated by R.F.C. Hull. Princeton: Princeton University Press.

———. 1990. "Psychologiczne podstawy wiary w duchy," translated by Jerzy Prokopiuk. In K. Jankowski. *Psychologia wierzeń religijnych.* Warszawa: Czytelnik.

————. 1991. *O psychologii i psychopatologii tzw. zjawisk tajemnych*, translated by Elżbieta Sadowska. Warszawa: Wydawnictwo Sen.

————. 1995. *Odpowiedź Hiobowi*, translated by Jerzy Prokopiuk. Warszawa: Wydawnictwo Ethos.

————. 1999. *Psychologia a alchemia*, translated by Robert Reszke. Warszawa: Wydawnictwo Wrota.

————. 2014. "A Psychological Approach to the Dogma of the Trinity." In *Psychology and Western Religion*, translated by R.F.C. Hull, 3–96. London, New York: Routledge.

Kelly, Edward F., and Emily Williams Kelly et al. 2010. *Irreducible Mind: Toward Psychology For the 21st Century*. Lanham, Boulder, New York, Toronto, Plymouth: Rowman & Littlefield Publishers.

Kępiński, Antoni. 1992. *Schizofrenia*. Kraków: Sagittarius.

Kocańda, Bogdan. 2004. *Posługa kapłana-egzorcysty. Duchowość, tożsamość, praktyka*. Kraków: Wydawnictwo "Bratni Zew."

Kołakowski, Leszek. 2000. *Główne nurty marksizmu. Rozwój*. Poznań: Wydawnictwo Zysk i S-ka.

Kościelniak, Krzysztof. 1999. *Złe duchy w Biblii i Koranie. Wpływ demonologii biblijnej na koraniczne koncepcje szatana w kontekście oddziaływań religii starożytnych*. Kraków: Wydawnictwo Unum.

Kratochvíl, Stanislav. 1996. *Hipnoza kliniczna*, translated by Marcela Czabak, and Andrzej Stanisław Piotrowski. Warszawa: Wydawnictwo KR.

Kuhn, Thomas S. 2012. *The Structure of Scientific Revolutions*. Chicago: University of Chicago Press.

Kutter, Peter. 1998. *Współczesna psychoanaliza. Psychologia procesów nieświadomych*, translated by Aleksandra Ubertowska. Gdańsk: Gdańskie Wydawnictwo Psychologiczne.

Lacan, Jacques. 1987. "Stadium zwierciadła jako czynnik kształtujący funkcję 'ja', w świetle doświadczenia psychoanalitycznego,' translated by J. W. Aleksandrowicz. *Psychoterapia*, issue 4 (63): 5–9. Kraków.

Laing, Ronald David. 2001. *The Divided Self: An Existential Study in Sanity and Madness*, London, New York: Routledge.

Langemeyer, Georg. 1995. *Antropologia teologiczna*, translated by Janina Fenrychowa. Kraków: Wydawnictwo M.

Langkammer, Hugolin. 1993. *Mały słownik biblijny*. Wrocław: Wydawnictwo św. Antoniego.

Laplanche, Jean, and Jean-Bertrand Pontalis. 2006. *The Language of Psychoanalysis*, translated by Donald Nicholson-Smith. London: Karnac Books.

Laszlo, Ervin. 2007. *Science and the Akashic Field. An Integral Theory of Everything*. Rochester: Inner Traditions.

Leeuw, Gerardus van der. 1997. *Fenomenologia religii*, translated by Jerzy Prokopiuk. Warszawa: Książka i Wiedza.

Levack, Brian P. 1991. *Polowanie na czarownice w epoce wczesnonowożytnej*, translated by Edward Rutkowski. Wrocław: Zakład Narodowy im. Ossolińskich.

Lévinas, Emmanuel. 1991. *Etyka i Nieskończony*, translated by Bogna Opolska–Kokoszka, Kraków: Wydawnictwo Naukowe Papieskiej Akademii Teologicznej.

Lévi-Strauss, Claude. 1966. *The Savage Mind*, edited by Julian Pitt-Rivers, and Ernest Gellner. Chicago, London: The University of Chicago Press.

Lowen, Alexander. 1997. *Narcissism: Denial of the True Self*. New York, London, Toronto, Sydney: Touchstone.

Madre, Philippe. 1999. *Boża miłość a dar uwalniania*, translated by Alina Liduchowska. Kraków: Wydawnictwo M.

Malinowski, Bronisław. 1984. "Wierzenia pierwotne i formy ustroju społecznego. Pogląd na genezę religii ze szczególnym uwzględnieniem totemizmu." In Bronisław Malinowski. *Dzieła*, vol.1. Warszawa: Wydawnictwo Naukowe PWN.

———. 1990. "O studiach Émile'a Durkheima," translated by D. Praszałowicz. In Bronisław Malinowski. *Dzieła*, vol. 1. Warszawa: Państwowe Wydawnictwo Naukowe.

Marcus Aurelius. 2018. "Exhortations to Himself." In Brad Inwood. *Stoicism: A Very Short Introduction.* Oxford: Oxford University Press.

Marx, Karl. 1982. *Critique of Hegel's 'Philosophy Of Right'*, translated by Annette Jolin, and Joseph O'Malley, edited by Joseph O'Malley. Cambridge: Cambridge University Press.

Maturana, Humberto R. and Varela, Francisco J. 1998. *The Tree of Knowledge: The Biological Roots of Human Understanding*, translated by Robert Paolucci. Boston and London: Shambhala.

Mauss, Marcel. 2001. *Socjologia i antropologia*, translated by Marcin Król, Krzysztof Pomian, and Jerzy Szacki. Warszawa: Państwowe Wydawnictwo Naukowe.

McTaggart, Lynne. 2008. *The Field Updated Ed: The Quest for the Secret Force of the Universe*. New York, London, Toronto, Sydney: Harper.

Meissner, William W. 1984. *Psychoanalysis and Religious Experience*. New Haven and London: Yale University Press.

Minuchin, Salvador, Bernice L. Rosman, and Lester Baker. 1978. *Psychosomatic Families. Anorexia Nervosa in Context*. Cambridge: Harvard University Press.

Moody, Raymond A. 2015. *Life After Life: The Bestselling Original Investigation That Revealed Near-Death Experiences*. New York: HarperOne.

Moore, Burness E., and Bernard D. Fine. 1996. *Słownik psychoanalizy*, translated by Ewa Modzelewska. Warszawa: Jacek Santorski & Co.

Morabito, Simone. 2011. *Psychiatra w piekle*. Kraków: AA.

Morrison, James. 2014. *DSM-5 Made Easy: The Clinician's Guide to Diagnosis*. New York, London: The Guilford Press.

Moskowitz, Andrew, and Gerhard Heim. 2011. "Eugen Bleuler's *Dementia Praecox or the Group of Schizophrenias* (1911): A Centenary Appreciation and Reconsideration." *Schizophrenia Bulletin*, vol. 37 (3), 471–479.

Musser, George. 2015. *Spooky Action at a Distance: The Phenomenon That Reimagines Space and Time--and What It Means for Black Holes, the Big Bang, and Theories of Everything*. New York: Scientific American.

Nicholas of Cusa. 1997. *O oświeconej niewiedzy*, translated by Ireneusz Kania. Kraków: Znak.

Nietzsche, Friedrich. 1968. *The Will to Power*, translated by Walter Kaufmann, and R. J. Hollingdale, edited by Walter Kaufmann. New York: Vintage Books.

———. 1989. *On the Genealogy of Morals and Ecce Homo*, edited by Walter Kaufmann, translated by Walter Kaufmann, and R. J. Hollingdale. New York: Vintage Books.

———. 1992. *Jutrzenka. Myśli o przesądach moralnych*, translated by Stanisław Wyrzykowski. Warszawa: Wydawnictwo BIS.

———. 2003. *Daybreak: Thoughts on the Prejudices of Morality*, translated by R. J. Hollingdale, edited by Maudemarie Clark, and Brian Leiter. Cambridge: Cambridge University Press.

———. 2004a. *Zmierzch bożyszcz, czyli jak filozofuje się młotem*, translated by Paweł Pieniążek. Kraków: "Zielona Sowa."

———. 2004b. *Ecce Homo: How One Becomes what One is & The Antichrist: a Curse on Christianity*, translated by Thomas Wayne. New York: Algora Publishing.

———. 2005. *The Anti-Christ, Ecce Homo, Twilight of the Idols, And Other Writings*, translated by Judith Norman, edited by Aaron Ridley and Judith Norman. Cambridge: Cambridge University Press.

———. 2017. "Beyond Good and Evil." In *The Essential Nietzsche: Beyond Good and Evil and The Genealogy of Morals*. New York: Chartwell Books.

Nijinsky, Vaslav. 2000. *Dziennik*, translated by Grzegorz Wiśniewski. Warszawa: "Iskry."

Ochorowicz, Julian. 1996. *Pierwsze zasady psychologii i inne pisma.* Warszawa: Wydawnictwo Naukowe PWN.

O'Connell, Erin. 2006. *Heraclitus and Derrida: Presocratic Deconstruction.* New York, Washington D.C. / Baltimore, Bern, Frankfurt am Mein, Berlin, Brussels, Vienna, Oxford: Peter Lang.

Ostrzycka, Anna, and Marek Rymuszko. 1989. *Nieuchwytna siła.* Warszawa: Oficyna Literatów "Rój."

———. 1994. *Powrót nieuchwytnej siły.* Warszawa: Wydawnictwo Fenomen.

Oświęcimski, Stefan. 1989. *Zeus daje tylko znak, Apollo wieszczy osobiście. Starożytne wróżbiarstwo greckie.* Wrocław: Zakład Narodowy im. Ossolińskich.

Otto, Rudolf. 1958. *The Idea of the Holy: An Inquiry Into the Non-rational Factor in the Idea of the Divine and Its Relation to the Rational*, translated by John W. Harvey. London, Oxford, New York: Oxford University Press.

Padgett, Jason, and Maureen Ann Seaberg. 2014. *Struck by Genius: How a Brain Injury Made Me a Mathematical Marvel.* New York: Houghton Mifflin Harcourt Publishing Company.

Pajor, Kazimierz. 2004. *Psychologia archetypów Junga.* Warszawa: Eneteia.

Pascal, Blaise. 2018. *Pensées*, translated by W.F. Trotter, edited by Susan L. Rattiner, and Lynne Rose Cannon. Mineola, New York: Dover Publications.

Pellegrin, Pierre. 2000. *Greek Thought: A Guide to Classical Knowledge*, translated by Catherine Porter, edited by Jacques Brunschwig and Geoffrey E. R. Lloyd. Cambridge, Massachusetts, London: The Belknap Press of Harvard University Press.

Pietras, Henryk. 2000. "Szatan a początek świata materialnego." In Henryk Pietras. *Demonologia w nauce ojców Kościoła*. Kraków: Wydawnictwo WAM.

*Pismo Święte Nowego testamentu i Psalmów*. 1991. Translated by The Benedictines of Tyniec. Warszawa: Pallottinum.

Plato. 1992. "Phaedo." In *The Trial and Death of Socrates: Four Dialogues*, translated by Benjamin Jowett, 55–128. New York: Dover Publications.

Plato. 1998. *Phaedrus*, translated by James H. Nichols Jr. Ithaca and London: Cornell University Press.

Plato. 2016. *Timaeus*. Translated and edited by Peter Kalkavage. Indianapolis, Cambridge: Hackett Publishing Company.

Plutarch. 2004. *The Life of Alexander the Great*, translated by John Dryden, edited by Arthur Hugh Clough. New York: The Modern Library.

Popper, Karl. 2000. *Knowledge and the Body-Mind Problem: In Defence of Interaction*, edited by M. A. Notturno. London, New York: Routledge.

Prątnicka, Wanda. 2007. *Opętani przez duchy. Egzorcyzmy w XXI stuleciu*. Gdynia: Wydawnictwo CENTRUM.

Pużyński, Stanisław, and Jacek Wciórka (eds.). 2000. *Klasyfikacja zaburzeń psychicznych i zaburzeń zachowania w ICD–10. Opisy kliniczne i wskazówki diagnostyczne*. Kraków – Warszawa: Uniwersyteckie Wydawnictwo Medyczna "Vesalius," Instytut Psychiatrii i Neurologii.

Quarantotto, Diana (ed.). 2018. *Aristotle's Physics Book I: A Systematic Exploration*. Cambridge: Cambridge University Press.

Reale, Giovanni. 1993. *Historia filozofii starożytnej*, vol.1, translated by Edward Iwo Zieliński. Lublin: KUL.

———. 1999. *Historia filozofii starożytnej*, vol.3, translated by Edward Iwo Zieliński. Lublin: KUL.

Reich, Wilhelm. 1961. *The Function of the Orgasm*, translated by Theodore P. Wolfe. New York: Noonday Press.

Rizzuto, Ana-María. 1990. "Freud," translated by Piotr Kołyszko. In Kazimierz Jankowski. *Psychologia wierzeń religijnych*. Warszawa: Czytelnik.

Rodewyk, Adolf. 1995. *Demoniczne opętanie dzisiaj. Fakty i interpretacje*, translated by Małgorzata Grzesik. Racibórz: R.A.F. Scriba.

Rops, Daniel. 1997. *Kościół pierwszych wieków*, translated by Kinga Ostrowska. Warszawa: PAX.

Rosenhan, David L., and Martin E. Seligman. 1994. *Psychopatologia*, translated by Danuta Golec, vol. 1. Warszawa: Polskie Towarzystwo Psychologiczne.

Rosińska, Zofia. 2002. *Freud*. Warszawa: Wiedza Powszechna.

Rusbridger, Richard. 2000. "Elements of the Oedipus Complex: Building up the Picture." *Oedipus Complex Today. The 3rd* Cracow International Psychoanalytical Symposium. Kraków.

Rycroft, Charles. 1995. *A Critical Dictionary of Psychoanalysis*. London: Penguin Books.

Sacks, Oliver. 1998. *Zobaczyć głos*, translated by Adam Małaczyński. Poznań: Wydawnictwo Zysk i S-ka.

Sadock, Benjamin James, and Virginia Alcott Sadock. 2008. *Kaplan & Sadock's Concise Textbook of Clinical Psychiatry.* Philadelphia: Wolters Kluwer/Lippincott Williams & Wilkins.

Samuels, Andrew, Bani Shorter, and Fred Plaut. 1986. *A Critical Dictionary of Jungian Analysis.* London, New York: Routledge.

Satir, Virginia, Richard Bandler, and John Grinder. 1976. *Changing with Families: A Book About Further Education for Being Human.* Palo Alto: Science and Behavior Books.

———. 1983. *Conjoint Family Therapy.* Palo Alto: Science and Behavior Books.

Scanlan, Michael, and Randall Cirner. 1999. *Uwalnianie ze złych mocy. Podstawy chrześcijańskiej walki duchowej,* translated by Kinga Maciuszak. Kraków: Wydawnictwo M.

Segal, Hanna. 1974. *Introduction to the work of Melanie Klein.* New York: Basic Books.

———. 2003. *Marzenie senne, wyobraźnia i sztuka,* translated by Paweł Dybel. Kraków: Universitas.

———. 2006. *Teoria Melanie Klein w praktyce klinicznej,* translated by Danuta Golec, Grażyna Rutkowska, and Anna Czownicka. Gdańsk: Gdańskie Wydawnictwo Psychologiczne.

Selye, Hans. 1960. *Stress życia,* translated by Jan W. *Guzek,* and Roman Rembiesa. Warszawa: Państwowy Zakład Wydawnictw Lekarskich.

Sheldrake, Rupert. 2009. *A New Science of Life.* London: Icon Books.

Sigmund, Georg (ed.). 2004. *Cztery głośne przypadki wypędzenia szatana,* translated by Zygmunt Sołek. Kraków: Wydawnictwo "Bratni Zew."

Spork. 2011. *Drugi kod. Epigenetyka, czyli jak możemy sterować własnymi genotypami,* translated by Viktor Grotowicz. Warszawa: W.A.B.

Stachowski, Ryszard. 1992. *The Mathematical Soul: An Antique Prototype of the Modern Mathematisation of Psychology.* Amsterdam, Atlanta: Rodopi.

Stanley, Barbara, Marc J. Gameroff, Venezia Michalsen, and J. John Mann. 2001. "Are Suicide Attempters Who Self-Mutilate a Unique Population?" *The American Journal of Psychiatry,* vol. 158, Issue 3 (March): 427–32.

Stefański, Lech Emfazy, and Michał Komar. 1996. *Od magii do psychotroniki czyli ars magica.* Warszawa: Bellona.

Symington, Neville. 1993. *Narcissism: A New Theory.* London: Karnac Books.

———. 1996. *The Making of a Psychotherapist.* London: Karnac Books.

Szasz, Thomas S. 1960. "The Myth of Mental Illness." *American Psychologist,* vol. 15(2), 113-18.

Szyjewski, Andrzej. 2000. *Religie Australii.* Kraków: Zakład Wydawniczy NOMOS.

———. 2001. *Etnologia religii.* Kraków: Zakład Wydawniczy NOMOS.

Tacey, David. 2012. *The Jung Reader.* London, New York: Routledge.

Taub-Bynum, E. B. 1984. *The Family Unconscious: An Invisible Bond.* Wheaton, Illinois: Quest Books.

Taylor, Christopher Charles Whiston (ed.). 2003. *From the Beginning to Plato.* London, New York: Routledge.

Teresa of Avila. 1921. *The Interior Castle, or The Mansions*, translated by The Benedictines of Stanbrook. London: Thomas Baker.

Tertullian. 2007. "On Fasting." In *The Ante-Nicene Fathers*, vol. IV, edited by Alexander Roberts, James Donaldson, and Arthur Cleveland Coxe, 102–15. New York: Cosimo.

Thomä, Helmut, and Horst Kächele. 1985. *Psychoanalytic Practice: 1 Principles*, translated by M. Wilson and D. Roseveare. Berlin, Heidelberg: Springer-Verlag.

Thomas Aquinas. 1999. *On Faith and Reason*, edited by Stephen F. Brown. Indianapolis, Cambridge: Hackett Publishing Company.

Trillat, Etienne. 1993. *Historia histerii*, translated by Zofia Podgórska–Klawe, and Elżbieta Jamrozik. Wrocław: Zakład Narodowy im. Ossolińskich.

Trotsky, Leon. 2005. *Literature and Revolution*, translated by Rose Strunsky, edited by William Keach. Chicago, Illinois: Haymarket Books.

Trzynadlowski, Jan (ed.). 1979. *Witelo—matematyk, fizyk, filozof.* Wrocław: Ossolineum.

Unterman, Alan. 2000. *Encyklopedia tradycji i legend żydowskich*, translated by Olga Zienkiewicz. Warszawa: Książka i Wiedza.

Üstün, T. Bedirhan, A. Bertelsen, H. Dilling, J. van Drimmelen, et al. 1999. *ICD–10 Zaburzenia psychiczne u osób dorosłych. Opisy przypadków*, translated by Waldemar *Koszewski*, and Maria *Bnińska*. Gdańsk: Medical Press.

Wadsworth, Barry J. 1998. *Teoria Piageta. Poznawczy i emocjonalny rozwój dziecka*, translated by Małgorzata Babiuch. Warszawa: Wydawnictwa Szkolne i Pedagogiczne.

Wciórka, Jacek. 2002a. "Schizofrenia, zaburzenia schizotypowe i schizoafektywne." In Adam Bilikiewicz, Stanisław Pużyński, Janusz Rybakowski, Jacek Wciórka, *Psychiatria*, vol. 2. Wrocław: Elsevier Urban & Partner.

———. 2002b. "Psychopatologia." In Adam Bilikiewicz, Stanisław Pużyński, Janusz Rybakowski, Jacek Wciórka, *Psychiatria*, vol. 1. Wrocław: Elsevier Urban & Partner.

Weber, Max. 1963. *The Sociology of Religion*. Boston: Beacon Press.

———. 1995. "Asceza i duch kapitalizmu," translated by Jerzy Prokopiuk, and Henryk Wandowski, In Max Weber. *Szkice z socjologii religii*. Warszawa: Książka i Wiedza.

Wegscheider-Cruse, Sharon, Kathy Higby, Ted Klontz, and Ann Rainey. 1995. *Family reconstruction: The Living Theater Model*. Palo Alto: Science and Behavior Books.

Welldon, Estela V. 2010. *Matka, madonna, dziwka. Idealizacja i poniżenie macierzyństwa*, translated by Danuta Golec. Warszawa: Oficina Infigenium.

West, Cameron. 2003. *Pierwsza osoba liczby mnogiej. Historia moich wielu osobowości*, translated by Tomasz Bieroń. Poznań: Wydawnictwo Zysk i S-ka.

Weyl, Hermann. 1997. *Symetria*, translated by Stefan Kulczycki. Warszawa: Prószyński i S-ka.

Whyte, Lancelot Law. 1960. *The Unconscious Before Freud*. New York: Basic Books.

Wilson, Walter T. 2011. *Philo of Alexandria: On Virtues: Introduction, Translation, and Commentary*, translated by Walter T. Wilson. Leiden: Brill.

Wink, Walter. 1984. *Naming the Powers: The Language of Power in the New Testament*. Philadelphia: Fortress Press.

Witelo. 1268. *De causa primariapaenitentiae in hominibus et de naturadaemonum*. Padua. http://scriptores.pl/en/efontes/.

Witelo. 2000. "O naturze demonów," translated by Bogdan Burliga, Alojzy Szlakiewicz. In Witelo. *O naturze demonów, Św. Anzelm z Cantenbury, O upadku diabła*. Gdańsk: Wydawnictwo "Niebiańskie Sfery."

Wittgenstein, Ludwig. 1978. *Philosophical Grammar*, edited by Rush Rhees, translated by Antony Kenny. Berkeley and Los Angeles: University of California Press.

Wizel, Adam. 2001. *Pamiętnik pacjentki*. Kraków: Towarzystwo Autorów i Wydawców Prac Naukowych "Universitas."

Wróbel, Jacek. 1984. "Znaczenia ukrywane przez kulturę i jednostkę i ich odbicie w języku chorych na schizofrenię." *Psychiatria Polska*, vol. XVIII, issue 3.

Wulff, David M. 1999. *Psychologia religii. Klasyczna i współczesna*, translated by Paweł Socha, Przemysław Jabłoński, and Małgorzata Sacha-Piekło. Warszawa: Wydawnictwa Szkolne i Pedagogiczne.

Žižek, Slavoj. 1989. *The Sublime Object of Ideology*. London, New York: Verso.

———. 1992. *Looking Awry: An Introduction to Jacques Lacan Through Popular Culture*. Cambridge, Massachusetts, London: The MIT Press.

———. 1997. *The Plague of Fantasies*. London, New York: Verso.

# Index

Page references for figures are italicized.

taboo, 104, 177, 189n11
Teresa of Avila, Saint, 173
Thomas Aquinas, Saint, 89–90, 92
thoughtform, 165
Tiamat, 177
tjurunga, 99n7
transference, 18n9, 71–72, 85n2, 200
transgenerational, 175, 178
Trotsky, Leon, 41

unconscious. *See* the unconscious
the unconscious, 14, 16, 18n9, 30, 31,
    47, 49–50, 53–54, 61n10, 62n21, 73,
    82, 84, 85n2, 85n4, 87, 90, 100n10,
    109, 130, 132, 138, 145, 159n28,
    160n37, 164, 170–72, 174, 176–78,
    180–81, 184, 189n12, 192, 195–96,
    199, 219n8

voodoo, 164

Weber, Max, 24, 60n6
Wegscheider-Cruse, Sharon, 175
Winnicott, Donald, 159n32
Witelo, 3–4
Wittgenstein, Ludwig, 128
Wizel, Adam, 103, 112, 115, 117,
    156n4

# About the Author

**Damian Janus** graduated from the faculties of psychology, philosophy and religious studies at the Jagiellonian University (Krakow, Poland) and has specializations in clinical psychology and psycho-oncology. He participated in training courses in Gestalt psychotherapy, bodywork, psychodynamic psychotherapy, and Lacanian psychoanalysis. He also completed trainings in family constellations. He worked in a psychiatric ward, mental health clinic, and addiction treatment clinic, and has a private psychotherapeutic practice. He has been working as an psychotherapist for almost twenty years. He is an academic lecturer. He is interested in physics and the history of science and technology.

www.ingramcontent.com/pod-product-compliance
Lightning Source LLC
Chambersburg PA
CBHW022308280326
41932CB00010B/1027